"It is always one genius or another who creates new ways of combining ideas to make them even more powerful, and therefore more helpful. This time Dr. Will Cole has done it with *Ketotarian*, which I predict will power a movement. I am jealous that I didn't think of it first, but so happy that such a brilliant mind, and more importantly, such a great doctor has done it and now will be available to everyone's benefit."

—Alejandro Junger, MD,
New York Times bestselling author
of *Clean Gut* and *Clean Eats*

"Dr. Will Cole has done the ketogenic diet the right way! This fresh, new spin on the keto diet is a great way to take your health to the next level. By combining the best of a plant-based diet and the best of the ketogenic diet, *Ketotarian* is both healing and delicious."

—Josh Axe, DNM, DC, CNS,
author of *Eat Dirt*

"This book is a game changer. If you want to know how to do a ketogenic diet and a plant based diet the right way, look no further."

—Frank Lipman, MD, *New York Times*
bestselling author of *The New Health Rules*

"Dr. Will Cole's *Ketotarian* is hands down the best way for anyone to go plant-based. All the food you need to eat is easily laid out for maximum nutrition and maximum healing—no more second guessing. It will be everything you need and more."

—Lauren Scruggs Kennedy, author, lifestyle
blogger, and entrepreneur

"For years, I struggled to find a way to feel balanced and healthy. Dr. Will Cole played a huge role in helping me find a way to re-boot my system and make me feel strong again, whether at home or on the road. Now, I'm back to feeling empowered and in control of my body, and I know that is in part because of the way Dr. Cole guided me down the path toward daily optimal health."

—Kathryn Budig, international yoga teacher
and author of *Aim True*

"Having been a vegan or vegaquarian for more than 23 years, I understand the true challenges of conscious eating and practical life. *Ketotarian* offers a simple healthful approach, grounded in credible science, to help you thrive and achieve optimal wellness. I'm hugely grateful that Dr. Will Cole is leading this paradigm shift for humanity and the planet."

—Christopher Gavigan, co-founder of
The Honest Company and
author of *Healthy Child Healthy World*

"Will Cole is one of the most knowledgeable functional medicine experts I've had the pleasure of working with. For those looking to experience big changes without any sense of deprivation, this book is a must-read."

—Liz Moody, author of *Glow Pops* and
senior food editor at mindbodygreen

"Dr. Will Cole shows us how to invest in ourselves through proper diet and nutrition. After all, health is wealth. What a beautiful way to take care of our future today."

—Kelly Rutherford, actress

"Dr. Cole is a thought leader in whole-person health and someone I respect and learn from. The combination of plants and fasting represents the solution to the health crisis in the Western world. This book teaches that less is more, and we should all follow suit."

—Joel Kahn MD, FACC,
author of _The Plant-Based Solution_

"When it comes to health, knowledge is power, and Dr. Cole operates from a place of arming his patients with all the information they need to optimize brain, metabolism, and hormones. He also understands that wellness exists on a spectrum, and that many women, in particular, are walking a fine line between 'health' and a diagnostic medical code—he provides the tools to coach your body back from the cliff's edge."

—Elise Loehnen, chief content officer, goop

"I couldn't be more pleased to see this daring attempt at bringing together the best of a plant-based approach with the plethora of health benefits that come from being in a state of nutritional ketosis. Here's hoping _Ketotarian_ catches on to shift people away from the SAD diet that's killing them!"

—Jimmy Moore, international bestselling
author of _Keto Clarity_ and _The Keto Cure_

"I am a big believer in there is not one meal intake that suits all, but with the Ketotarian diet, Dr. Cole is successfully able to connect those looking to reduce inflammation, improve systematic brain function and harmonize one's hormonal state with incredible tasty and colorfully rich foods."

—Dan Churchill, international chef
and author of _DudeFood_

"Dr. Cole's new book is highly informative, yet easy to understand when it comes to what we should be eating and how to combat issues you might be facing. It's very important for my clients to know the 'why' behind how certain foods can affect them, and I believe this book gives great insight into solving some of those unanswered questions."

—Nikki Sharp, wellness expert and
author of _The 5-Day Real Food Detox_

"Burning ketones has fascinating health effects that get obscured by concerns of too much meat. I love this book because I have wondered—how the heck can you do a smart, healthy, plant-based keto diet in the real world?! Awesome to see my pal Dr. Will Cole deliver the delicious, nutritious answer!"

—Drew Ramsey, MD,
Assistant Clinical Professor of Psychiatry
Columbia University, New York, New York

"I will be using Dr. Cole's book as a resource for patients with metabolic conditions such as obesity, Type 1 and Type 2 diabetes, neurologic and pain conditions where we are trying to reduce inflammation and decrease pain, and patients with musculoskeletal related autoimmune conditions. Dr. Cole does an excellent job of explaining complex biochemistry, physiology and the most current research, while at the same time delivering a plan that is clear cut and straightforward to follow. If you are struggling to lose weight or improve your health with a standard plant-based or a ketogenic diet, _Ketotarian_ is definitely for you."

—Carrie Diulus, MD,
Orthopaedic Spine Surgeon; Medical Director,
Crystal Clinic Spine Wellness Center;
thriving type 1 diabetic

keto·tarian

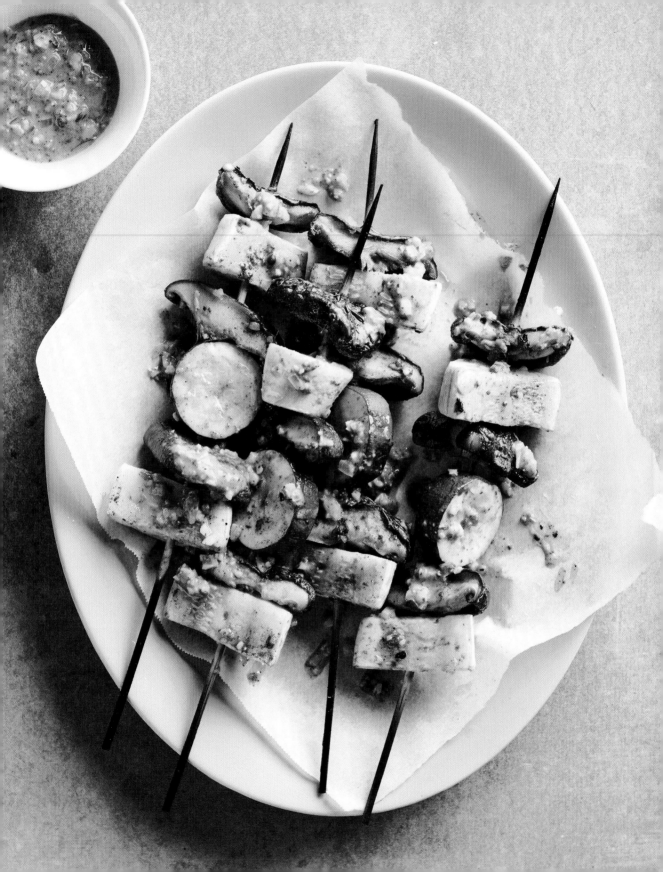

keto·tarian

the (mostly) plant-based plan to burn fat,
boost your energy, crush your cravings,
and calm inflammation

Dr. Will Cole

AVERY

an imprint of Penguin Random House
New York

AVERY

an imprint of Penguin Random House LLC
375 Hudson Street
New York, New York 10014

Most Avery books are available at special quantity discounts
for bulk purchase for sales promotions, premiums, fund-raising,
and educational needs. Special books or book excerpts
also can be created to fit specific needs. For details,
write SpecialMarkets@penguinrandomhouse.com.

ISBN 9780525537175
ebook ISBN: 9780525537182

Printed in the United States of America
3 5 7 9 10 8 6 4

Book design by Ashley Tucker

contents

introduction

the ketotarian manifesto

ketotarian [kee-toe-tair-ee-uhn]

noun

A ketogenic plant-based rock star.

adjective

1   The amalgamation of delicious healthy fats and vegetable meals to optimize your metabolism, brain, hormones and overall health.
2   Switching your metabolism from burning sugar to burning fat—that is, freedom from food cravings.

This is the manifesto for a new breed of health seekers and eaters. The pages you are reading are for anyone who wants to ditch dieting for good and actually get healthy. This book is the new manual to cut through food confusion and find out what to eat and what not to eat to lose weight, crush cravings, calm inflammation, and achieve optimal energy levels.

We are over trying another unsustainable fad diet only to gain it all back (and then some). Let's get healthy to lose weight, instead of trying to lose weight to get healthy. Sustainable weight loss should be a natural by-product of regained, radiant health.

These days we have an overwhelming amount of information at our fingertips. The double-edged sword of Dr. Google is that he can both educate us about our health and yet suffocate us with conflicting information on what the heck we should eat, an endless vortex of conflicting information. Dr. Google is one fickle, confused guy.

So what *is* the best way to your optimal health? Should you focus on high-meat diets like the paleo or Atkins ways of eating, or will they clog your arteries and make you fat? Maybe becoming a vegan or vegetarian is the answer, consuming only plant food. But will that deprive your body of nutrients like B vitamins and iron, and don't those diets focus heavily on soy and grains, and isn't *that* unhealthy?

Ketotarian will show you the clear path of exactly how to use food as medicine and optimize every system in your body. Your brain, hormones, and metabolism will thrive in the Ketotarian state.

You may be thinking that's a bold statement, but as a leading functional medicine practitioner, rated as one of the top in the country, I have seen thousands of patients from around the world. I have seen what works and what doesn't when it comes to the foods we eat. And I've distilled my years of clinical experience, using the power of delicious food medicine, in the pages of this book.

You may have heard of the ketogenic diet. This low-carbohydrate, moderate-protein, high-fat way of eating has taken the wellness world by storm. The ketogenic diet promises to shift your metabolism into a fat-burning powerhouse, allowing you to lose stubborn weight that you may have been holding on to for years. The ketogenic diet promises not only weight loss but also a way to improve your brain function and decrease chronic inflammation, the root factor to just about every chronic health problem we face today.

The problem is that the average ketogenic dieter is eating pounds of processed meats, bacon, beef, cheese, and dairy from factory-farmed animals. These foods are loaded with antibiotics and hormones, but many keto dieters believe it's fine because it's "low-carb, high-fat." The conventional ketogenic diet also allows you to have sugar-free, artificial sweeteners like aspartame, sucralose, and diet drinks all in the name of being "low carb." These sweeteners are linked to triggering a whole array of health problems, but as long as it's low-carb, it's OK on the average ketogenic diet. As long as it fits the right macronutrient ratio, your average keto dieter will eat it. Because of this hyperfocus on macronutrients over food quality, many people on the ketogenic diet begin to fear and avoid vegetables because of their carbohydrate content. This is a major issue I have with the standard ketogenic approach.

Then there are the vegan and vegetarian diets. Typically, these are the antithesis of the ketogenic diet: low-fat and high-carb. Advocates of this way of eating tell us that avoiding animal products like meat and dairy not only will reverse and prevent disease and protect our heart health but is also good for the planet. Opting for plants instead of meat is said to reduce our carbon footprint and protect against climate change. Contrary to the ketogenic diet, vegans and vegetarians often encourage us to eat a low-fat, moderate-plant-protein, high-carbohydrate diet—the polar opposite of a ketogenic approach to eating.

The problem I find in vegan and vegetarian patients is that most of them are actually carbatarians, living on bread, pasta, beans, and vegan sweets, all in the name of living green. If they aren't bread heads, they are depending too heavily on soy for their protein, which is typically genetically modified and always high in estrogens. I see many vegans and vegetarians with wrecked digestion and their overall health declining, clinging to their zealous belief that this is the way people should eat and live.

It's time to dump diet dogma and food fads for good. What really works—and what really doesn't—for your health?

Ketotarian marries the best of low-carb diets and a plant-based way of eating, while avoiding the common pitfalls that I have seen countless well-intentioned people make with both these diets. The Ketotarian way of eating brings together healthy plant-based fats, clean protein, and the rich, vibrant colors of nutrient-dense vegetables.

It's time to dump diet dogma and food fads for good. What really works—and what really doesn't—for your health?

the age of inflammation

A storm is brewing in our society: the storm of inflammation. At least fifty million Americans have an autoimmune condition, millions more are somewhere on the autoimmune-inflammation spectrum, someone has a heart attack every thirty-four seconds, and a shocking one in two men and one in three women will get cancer. Sadly, these numbers have only been increasing. Just because something is common doesn't make it normal. This level of disease is ubiquitous, but it is certainly not normal. All of these conditions have one thing in common: inflammation.

When your immune system is balanced, its inflammatory response will save your life. Injuries and infections are healed with the power of balanced, calm inflammation levels. Conversely, when your immune system is unbalanced, it is a perpetual fire, affecting every cell of your body.

Imbalance breeds destruction. Just as the earth's climate is changing, an unbalanced immune system is turning against itself in the form of chronic disease and autoimmunity, in which the body's defense system goes into overdrive, attacking healthy systems unnecessarily.

In addition, nearly 20 percent of adults have a diagnosable mental disorder.[1] Depression, which is now believed to be an inflammatory condition, is the leading cause of disability worldwide. Anxiety disorders affect more than forty million Americans, and Alzheimer's disease is the sixth leading cause of death in the United States. In fact, one report found that since 1979, deaths due to brain disease have increased by 66 percent in men and a whopping 92 percent in women.[2] Autism and autism spectrum disorders (ASDs) have skyrocketed over a short period of time. In 1970, an estimated 1 in 10,000 children were found to be autistic; in 1995 it was 1 in 500, and in 2001 it became 1 in 250. Today, at least 1 in 68 children are diagnosed as autistic. An estimated 1 in 5 American children ages 3 to 17 (about fifteen million kids) have a diagnosable mental, emotional, or behavioral disorder. Research has shown that serious depression is worsening among teens, especially girls, and the suicide rate among girls reached a forty-year high recently, according to the Centers for Disease Control and Prevention (CDC).[3]

The United States spends more on health care than the next ten top-spending countries *combined*.[4] And even though we spend trillions of dollars, we rank among the last of all industrialized nations when it comes to living long, healthy lives. According to the *Journal of the American Medical Association (JAMA)*, out of thirteen industrialized nations the United States is one of the worst when it comes to years of life lost for adults and infant mortality rates.[5] Another report, this one from the United Health Foundation, showed similar findings. The report compared the U.S. life expectancy with that of thirty-five other countries. Despite spending more on health care per capita, the United States ranked twenty-seventh against comparable nations.[6]

A shocking 81 percent of Americans take at least one medication a day. Prescription drugs are now said to kill more people than heroin and cocaine combined.[7]

According to *JAMA*,[8] more than one hundred thousand people die each year from the proper use of prescription drugs: not from overdosing or taking the wrong drug but from the side effects of the "right drug."[9]

The multibillion-dollar pharmaceutical industry is only expected to continually grow. In functional medicine, we're not anti-medication. We recognize that many people are alive because of medications, and advancements in modern medicine have brought us lifesaving procedures, especially in emergency care. We just ask the question: What is our most effective option that causes the least amount of side effects? For some, a medication may fit this logical criterion. But in many cases, pharmaceuticals do not, yet that is often the only option presented.

your dna is not your destiny

Research has shown that over 90 percent of our longevity is determined by the choices we make—not our genetics. Sure, people can have a genetic predisposition for certain diseases (most of us do), but that particular gene may not be expressed if it's not triggered by these epigenetic, lifestyle factors.

Research like the Okinawa study has shown that there is no reason why most of us can't live for about one hundred disease-free, healthy years. It's the interaction between our genes and our environment that determines our health. The foods we eat or don't eat, our stress levels, sleep, activity, and exposure to toxins are constantly and dynamically instructing our genetic expression. This is a revolutionary message of health empowerment and responsibility.

the best medicine is at the end of our forks

With the Hippocratic advice to "let food be thy medicine, and medicine thy food," how far have we strayed that the words of the founder of modern medicine can actually be threatening to conventional medicine?

Today medical schools in the United States offer, on average, only about nineteen hours of nutrition education over four years of medical school.[10] Only 29 percent of U.S. medical schools offer med students the recommended twenty-five hours of nutrition education.[11] A study in the *International Journal of Adolescent Medicine and Health* assessed the basic nutrition and health knowledge of medical school graduates entering a pediatric residency program and found that, on average, they answered only 52 percent of the eighteen questions correctly.[12] In short, most mainstream doctors would fail nutrition. So if you were wondering why someone in functional medicine, outside conventional medicine, is writing a book on how to use food for optimal health, this is why.

Expecting health guidance from mainstream medicine is akin to getting gardening advice from a mechanic. You can't expect someone who wasn't properly trained in a field to give sound advice. Brilliant physicians in the mainstream model of care are trained to diagnose a disease and match it with a corresponding pharmaceutical drug. This medicinal matching game works sometimes, but often it leaves the patient with nothing but a growing prescription list and growing health problems.

With the strong influence that the pharmaceutical industry has on government and conventional medical policy, it's no secret that using foods to heal the body is not a priority of mainstream medicine. You only need to eat hospital food once to know this truth. Even more, under current laws it is illegal to say that foods can heal. That's right. The words *treat, cure,* and *prevent* are in effect owned by the Food and Drug Administration (FDA) and the pharmaceutical industry and can be used in the health care setting only when talking about medications. This is the Orwellian world we live in today; health problems are on the rise even though we spend more on health care than ever, and getting healthy is considered radical and often labeled as quackery.

But with the ubiquity of chronic inflammation, it's important to know where your inflammation levels are and what's fueling them.

The most common source of the chronic inflammation we see today is the foods we eat, namely sugar, and foods that turn into sugar, namely processed, refined carbohydrates.

The definition of doing the same thing repeatedly is insanity. I'm not calling you insane! As a culture, we should look around at the unintended consequences of our collective decisions. We need to do something different to see different results.

sugar vs. fat:
what are you fueling your body with?

The standard Western diet today is centered on many forms of the very same thing: sugar.

From the refined carbohydrates of junk foods to breads, pastas, fruit, and juices, sugar makes up most of what we're eating. But is it the best form of energy for your brain, metabolism, and body?

Most people struggling with health problems like fatigue, hormone imbalances, immune dysfunctions, and brain and metabolic issues are in sugar-burning mode: going from one sugary or grain-based meal to the next, becoming "hangry" (*hungry* and *angry*'s grumpy spawn) if they don't get their fix. Even healthy, clean eaters can be stuck on this blood sugar roller coaster.

On the other hand, a healthy ketogenic diet—where fat, not sugar, is your primary source of energy—has been shown to do some remarkable things for our brain health. And healthy fats are a slow, sustainable form of energy, unlike the sugary roller coaster many find themselves on. After all, biology knows best: as babies, we were all born relying on fat in the form of breast milk for brain development and energy.

Bottom line: making our brain and body work properly requires a lot of energy. And from a biological and evolutionary perspective, the most sustainable form of energy for optimal brain health is good fats.

A ketogenic state is the true natural state for the human body. In the pages that follow, you will learn how to reprogram your metabolism. Like a factory reset, you can shift from sugar-burning back to fat-burning, the way your body was designed to operate.

Fat, in terms of energy to your body, is like a log on a fire, slow-burning and long-lasting. The typical pick-me-up foods of grains and sugar are like kindling, a quick burst of intense flame that dies out, leaving behind nothing but smoke. This means that becoming fat- or keto-adapted not only gives you sustainable energy throughout the day for your brain and metabolism but also crushes food cravings. Insatiable, intense food cravings are one of the top reasons most diets fail. This is not an issue for the Ketotarian.

So instead of focusing on foods that offer only a quick burst of energy but leave you crashing later, let's focus on how to nourish your body with good food medicine. You can start regaining energy today just by following the Ketotarian plan. In addition to the healthy fats you need for fuel, I have also included the world's best foods to fight fatigue and rev up your metabolism. This, my friend, is your energy rehab plan.

When it comes to dieting, willpower and calorie counting fail us most of the time. You need to dump dieting and get healthy. You need to ditch dieting and shift your metabolism to a fat-burning state. Tap into your body's full metabolic potential. By becoming a keto-adapted powerhouse, you will transcend insatiable cravings and the misery that comes with fad dieting in a sugar-burning state. As a Ketotarian, you will be eating filling foods, and you will be satisfied. This makes Ketotarian the anti-diet: a sustainable and realistic lifestyle.

Ketotarian includes the brain-boosting, fat-burning, hormone-healing, energizing benefits of a ketogenic diet without falling prey to inflammatory conventional meat that can be hard to digest and dairy that many people don't tolerate.

The Ketotarian way of living also reaps the many benefits of a plant-based diet without depending on carbs for short-lived energy. Let's get off the blood sugar roller coaster and start feeling fantastic. The plant-based nature of Ketotarian calms inflammation levels, aids in cleansing detoxification pathways, and feeds a healthy gut microbiome—all imperative for your optimal wellness.

We'll review the latest, cutting-edge research-based reasons why this is the most effective way to eat for living a long, healthy life. I will also share with you my favorite Ketotarian recipes that are both simple and delicious. You will know exactly what to eat to become a plant-based, ketogenic fat-burning machine so that you can feel and look your best.

the best of both worlds

Because Ketotarian is the best of both the ketogenic and plant-based worlds, it is meant for anyone and everyone. By eating the Ketotarian way you will get to experience satisfying and delicious ketogenic meals that are:

- **Plant-based** (most recipes are vegan or vegetarian)

- **Paleo/primal-friendly** (Ketotarian is naturally legume, dairy, gluten, and grain free and all real foods)

- **Autoimmune-friendly** (autoimmune protocol, AIP) (many recipes are free of nuts, nightshades, and eggs; all are free of grains and dairy)

This unique, fresh way of eating and living is meant for anyone who wants to lose weight, overcome cravings, regain energy, or decrease inflammation levels. If you've been confused and frustrated about what the heck to eat, look no further.

food peace

Maybe I'm a sucker for optimism, but in the world that we are living in today, can't we come together over what we have in common, yet accept and even celebrate our differences? Let's start in the kitchen and at the dinner table.

Ketotarian unifies all that is great with being plant-based and ketogenic. This is both sustainable and healing to you and the world we live in.

For me, Ketotarian goes much deeper than food—it's about freedom. Freedom from food that doesn't serve you or make you feel good. Freedom from insatiable cravings. Freedom from brain fog and fatigue. Freedom from unsustainable yo-yo dieting and rules. Freedom from the shame surrounding food. Body and food peace. This is a life-changing paradigm shift. Instead of a dieting consciousness, with shame and guilt, we are focused on feeling freaking fantastic. Knowing what makes your body thrive and what doesn't is true food freedom.

Let's start a revolution. Are you with me?

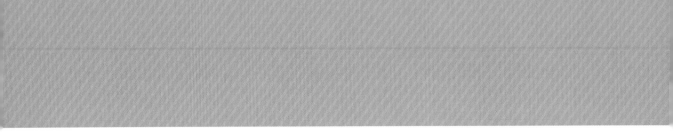

1

the ketogenic diet
(For Better and Worse)

OK, let's start with the basics. A ketogenic diet is a low-carbohydrate, high-fat (LCHF) diet, but what does that even mean? Well, let's start with the basics. First of all, not all low-carb diets are ketogenic. By using a specific ratio of macronutrients—high fats, moderate proteins, and low carbohydrates—you can shift your body into a fat-burning state known as ketosis.

keto principle #1: shift from sugar to fat to fuel your body more powerfully

Americans eat an average of 765 grams of sugar every five days—and much of it is hidden, added where you'd least expect it, or going by a different name. Compare that number to the 45 grams of sugar Americans ate back in 1822 over the same time period. Today the average American eats and drinks around 130 pounds of added sugar every year, adding up to an astounding 3,550 pounds in a lifetime. That's equal to eating 1.7 million Skittles or an industrial-sized Dumpster full of sugar. Dang, that's a lot of sugar, y'all.

Most people walking around today are burning carbohydrates (sugar) for their energy. Breaking down carbs into glucose is the simplest energy source, and insulin is there to help carry the glucose around your bloodstream throughout your body. And because high blood sugar is toxic, it is your body's priority to use the sugar "kindling" whenever it is around. The sugar your body doesn't burn is stored as fat around your liver and stomach and as circulating fat (triglycerides).

But as proponents of keto eating can attest, there *is* another way. Instead of burning sugar, burning fat is a more efficient fuel source for your metabolism. When you lower your carbohydrates, it lowers your blood sugar and insulin levels. As insulin levels normalize and energy is needed, fatty acids flow from the fat cells into the bloodstream and are metabolized by your body in a process called beta-oxidation.

The result of beta-oxidation is a molecule called acetyl-CoA, and as more fatty acids are released and metabolized, acetyl-CoA levels in the cells rise. This process causes a metabolic *feedback loop*, which tells your liver cells to use acetyl-CoA for ketogenesis, or the making of ketone bodies.

The liver then puts the ketone bodies into your bloodstream and fuels your body. Your brain can also use ketones as an alternative fuel source when blood levels are high enough to cross the blood-brain barrier, making ketones a brain superfood!

The keto diet isn't about starving your body of food—it's about allowing your body to be in a better metabolic state. Think of ketosis as converting your metabolism from a gasoline-burning to a hybrid engine, using fuel more efficiently.

There are three major types of ketone bodies that are in our bloodstream when we are in ketosis:

- **Acetoacetate (AcAc) is created first.**

- **Beta-hydroxybutyrate (BHB) is created from acetoacetate.**

- **Acetone (BrAce) is also created from acetoacetate.**

When blood sugar and insulin levels are low and healthy, ketones supply most of the energy required by your brain and body, becoming the primary source of fuel for your energy.

In the ketogenic state, ketones in the bloodstream will range between 0.5 and 5 mmol (millimolar concentration) depending on the amount of protein and carbo-hydrates that you eat. Welcome to nutritional ketosis, the metabolic promised land.

THE HEALTH BENEFITS OF KETOSIS

Nutritional ketosis has been shown to have many promising health applications. The following are some of the main benefits of a ketogenic state:

- **Weight loss**

- **Increased energy**

- Mental clarity

- Better blood pressure

- Improved acne and skin problems

- Lower inflammation throughout the body

- Curbed food cravings

- Reduced (if not eliminated) seizures in most people with epilepsy

- Lowered risk of some cancers

- Reversed or improved symptoms of polycystic ovary syndrome (PCOS)

- Improved (if not reversed) type 2 diabetes

We'll go over these health benefits, and others, in detail later on. But let's not get ahead of ourselves.

A healthy ketogenic lifestyle can be a way of taking back control of your body—not living for the next meal or having dips and lows in energy through the day but enjoying consistent energy and improved health.

IF YOU'RE HANGRY AND YOU KNOW IT, RAISE YOUR HAND

A ketogenic state is about metabolic efficiency. Like a hybrid vehicle, someone in nutritional ketosis burns primarily fat as their fuel. Being fat-adapted is a slow-burning and more sustainable way of living and eating. So basically, my Toyota Prius and my metabolism both run smoothly for a long time without having to fill up.

Relying on a sugar burn is akin to burning dirty fossil fuel. You need to fill up quickly or you'll run on empty, and it leaves behind all kinds of inflammatory pollution.

In addition to having to fill up quickly when you are depending on carbs and sugar for energy, it's also bad for your health. A staggering 50 percent of us are now either prediabetic or have full-blown type 2 diabetes. No, that is not a typo; one out of two of us has some serious blood sugar problems, making a condition that was once a rarity sadly commonplace. But just because something is common doesn't mean it's normal.

Our blood sugar problems are a modern phenomenon, born out of the mismatch between our DNA, unchanged for thousands of years, and the sugary, stressed-out, toxic world around us. The blood sugar roller coaster we experience each day is anything but normal. Blood sugar, just like your hormones, immune system, and gut bacteria, is subject to the Goldilocks principle: not too high, not too low, but just right.

Insulin Resistance Is at the Core of Blood Sugar Problems

Most of the blood sugar problems we see today are due to one thing: insulin resistance. Varying degrees of this hormonal imbalance wreak havoc on our health. Insulin is a hormone that instructs our body's cells to absorb blood sugar (glucose) and convert it into energy, and it also tells our cells to absorb glucose to convert it into body fat. With insulin resistance, your cell receptor sites are blunted and blocked because of inflammation or toxins, so the message is not received. This causes the body to make even more insulin to compensate, creating a vicious cycle. The result is excess body fat, coupled with reduced muscle mass. This not only makes you feel miserable but can lead to diabetes, which is one of the leading causes of heart attacks and strokes.

All foods stimulate insulin production to some extent. But the main food culprits are sugar and carbs (and to a lesser degree protein)—they're the key drivers of insulin spikes. If you eat healthy fats but don't limit your carbs and even your protein, your insulin and glucose levels can still be too high, and you won't reap the benefits of keto eating.

keto principle #2: fat is your friend

Fats have been controversial in the past, but they are finally, albeit slowly, being vindicated as essential for our health and not the disease-promoting, artery-clogging villain we were told they were.

For a long time, there was an endless barrage of misinformation and propaganda against eating fat. Although old belief systems die hard, we know now that

signs that your blood sugar has gone awry

So how do you know if you have a blood sugar problem? If more than one of these is true for you, I suggest getting your blood sugar levels checked:

- You crave sweets or breads and pastries . . . like, a lot.
- Eating sweets doesn't relieve your sugar cravings.
- You become irritable and "hangry" if you miss a meal.
- You find yourself needing caffeine to get through the day.
- You become light-headed if you miss a meal.
- Eating makes you exhausted and in need of a nap.

- It's difficult for you to lose weight.
- You feel weak, shaky, or jittery pretty frequently,
- You have to pee a lot.
- You get agitated, easily upset, or nervous.
- Your memory is not what it used to be.
- Your vision is blurry.
- Your waist is equal to or larger than your hips.
- You have a low sex drive.
- You're always thirsty.

You don't have to settle for these symptoms and the roller coaster of blood sugar highs and lows. That's what this book is all about. How can you be a lean (and green!) fat-burning machine.

I run the following lab tests on my patients to assess their blood sugar balance and check for insulin resistance:

- Serum insulin (optimal range: <3 ulU/mL)
- C-peptide (optimal range: 0.8 to 3.1 ng/mL)
- Fasting blood sugar (optimal range: 70 to 90 mg/dL)
- Hgb A1C (optimal range: <5.3 percent)
- Triglycerides (optimal range: <100 mg/dL)
- HDL (optimal range: 59 to 100 mg/dL)

cholesterol and saturated fats do not cause heart disease. Let's bust the fat myths and set the record straight once and for all!

Eating healthy fats like coconut, avocado, olive oil, and ghee with vegetables allows your body to better utilize the fat-soluble vitamins. Those healthy fats often contain fat-soluble vitamins like A, D, E, and K2, allowing your body to better absorb those nutrients. So eating fats with each of your meals will benefit your body's ability to absorb nutrients from your food.

Healthy fats are also essential for your cellular health. The foundation on which your body is formed needs these fats to build healthy cell membranes. Don't take this personally, but your brain is your fattest body part, made up of around 60 percent fat. Before you punch me, it's not just you, we are all fat-heads since birth, coming out of the womb relying on fat in the form of breast milk for brain development and energy.[13] Even if you weren't breast-fed, MCT, DHA, and ARA fats are added to formula to mimic breast milk!

> Healthy fats are essential for your cellular health. The foundation on which your body is formed needs these fats to build healthy cell membranes.

Healthy fats also aid in balancing your hormones. Cell communication is key in hormone health, and by eating a diet in healthy fats you are building up the pathways of communication throughout your body, making it easier for your hormones to convert and get where they need to be, helping you be hormonally balanced, which is needed for your mood, metabolism, and weight.

Because our cells, hormones, and brain depend on fats for optimal functioning, we are in effect starving them when we eat a low-fat diet long term.

The whole premise of the ketogenic diet is to have a more balanced energy source by relying on ketones over glucose for energy. By lowering your blood sugar and insulin to healthy levels and raising ketones to the nutritional ketosis range, you are maintaining healthy stress hormones like cortisol. This further balances inflammation and lowers stress on your immune system.

HEALTHY AND UNHEALTHY FATS

With all this focus on fat, it's essential to understand the difference between healthy and unhealthy fats. Some fats are essential for health, while others can fuel oxidative stress or inflammation and put a serious strain on your health. There are four different types of fat: monounsaturated fats, polyunsaturated fats, trans fats, and saturated fats.

Monounsaturated fats (MUFAs)—These fats are liquid at room temperature but become hard and solid when put in the fridge or are cooled. Olive oil, avocado oil, and seed and nut oils fall into this category. These oils can contribute to heart health and healthy cholesterol, reduced risk of stroke, improved insulin resistance, and reduced belly fat, among other benefits. For a healthy ketogenic diet centered on healthy fats, these are a simple staple to keep in your arsenal of foods.

Polyunsaturated fats (PUFAs)—Here's where many people get confused. While polyunsaturated fats found in fatty fish like sardines, salmon, and mackerel, as well as seeds and nuts such as flaxseeds and walnuts, are good for you, some other oils in this category are not great at all and can actually be very harmful to your health. The ones to avoid are canola oil, soybean oil, safflower oil, and vegetable oils. The difference here is that one is a natural polyunsaturated oil (like omega oils) and the other is a highly processed polyunsaturated fat (like vegetable and canola oils). While natural polyunsaturated oils can improve healthy cholesterol levels and calm inflammation, processed, refined ones do the exact opposite, fueling inflammation and messing up your lipids. Avoid the refined kinds whenever possible.

Trans fats—These are the fats your doctor, mother, and Facebook friends have all warned you about. Altering the chemical makeup of fats and adding hydrogen (thus the name *partially hydrogenated oil*) increases the shelf life of the fat—and the dangers, too. This is the type of fat that raises your LDL cholesterol and lowers your HDL cholesterol, which can lead to heart disease. If you pick up processed, packaged food in a grocery store and read the label, you will often see "partially hydrogenated oil." It's found in a variety of foods including margarine and creamers, and in baked goods like cookies, cakes, and potato chips. It's cheaper and has a more stable shelf life so it's used frequently—unfortunately, at the cost of your health. Trans fat (along with polyunsaturated fats) is also used in fryers in restaurants and fast-food chains.

Avoid this fat entirely. If you aren't sure what oil it is when you are eating out, ask. Pick up the labels and read. Be your own health advocate and avoid these fats that can and will hurt your health.

Saturated fats (SFAs)—Misunderstood and wrongly accused of being a culprit of heart disease, these are, in fact, a necessity for healthy immune function, hormone health, cellular health, and brain health. Examples of saturated fats are grass-fed butter, ghee (clarified butter), coconut oil, eggs, and meats. These fats actually can bring up healthy HDL cholesterol levels. Unlike monounsaturated oils, these are solid at room temperatures.

The studies that naysayers often cite to vilify saturated fats do not link eating more saturated fat to heart disease—rather, they link it to increasing cholesterol numbers.

The reality is, total cholesterol is a poor predictor for assessing heart attack and stroke risk. Studies have found that there might be no association between high total cholesterol and heart attack and stroke risk.[1]

It is very interesting that the fat-averse are still suggesting that we switch from using saturated fats like coconut oil to polyunsaturated fats like corn and vegetable oil. One source that they cite is the Minnesota Coronary Experiment, which is decades old. A recent reevaluation of the data published in the *British Medical Journal* found that study participants who swapped saturated fats for polyunsaturated corn oil had a 22 percent increased risk of death for every 30 points their cholesterol went down![2] Better predictors for heart attack and stroke risks are high inflammation markers like C-reactive protein (CRP) and homocysteine, low HDL ("good" cholesterol), high triglycerides, and high small dense LDL protein carriers. The other LDL subtype is the large buoyant particles, the nonoxidized, noninflamed LDL particles, which are protective just like HDL.

Researchers have found that high-fat diets containing healthy, real-food saturated fats like coconut raised HDL, lowering triglycerides and small LDL cholesterol particles.[3] Pacific Islanders who consumed a majority of their calories from healthy saturated fats raised their total cholesterol, mainly from their "good" HDL rising.[4] Another meta-analysis published in the *British Medical Journal* found no association between increased saturated fat intake and heart attack, stroke, and death risk.[5]

A randomized control trial published in the *American Journal of Clinical Nutrition* found a diet rich in fats, including a high percentage of calories from saturated fats, actually lowered cardiometabolic risk factors: HDL came up, triglycerides came down, insulin sensitivity improved, and blood sugar was lowered.[6]

The context and quality of a total cholesterol panel is so much more important than looking at a total cholesterol above 200 and deeming it "bad." It may be or may not be. The research shows that saturated fats like coconut oil seem to improve the quality of cholesterol while also increasing the quantity.

A growing number of studies show similar results:[7] that lowering dietary saturated fat and cholesterol did not decrease heart attacks. The problem with saturated fats like coconut oil occurs when people eat them with refined grains (which turn into sugar) such as breads and pasta or sugary foods. This "mixed meal" combination amplifies the inflammation of sugar. So, if you're not going to eat vegetables and avoid carby junk foods, I suggest limiting your saturated fat intake and always focusing on quality, real-food (and organic when possible) sources.

five ways to go keto

Everyone's health and needs are different, but the ketogenic diet can be applied using the following methods:

STANDARD KETOGENIC DIET (SKD)

The SKD is the most common and popular choice for those living a ketogenic lifestyle. This method focuses on a very-low-carb, moderate-protein, and high-fat diet. The original definition of the ketogenic diet was based on this premise.

This version is typically most effective and maintainable. Most often, this diet consists of a ratio of 75 percent healthy fats, 20 percent protein, and 5 percent carbohydrates.

HIGH-PROTEIN KETOGENIC DIET

The high-protein ketogenic diet is the same as the SKD except that it allows for a higher amount of protein—around 10 to 15 percent more protein, accompanied by a reduction of healthy fats by the same amount.

The ratios can be composed of two options; 60 percent fats, 35 percent protein, and 5 percent carbohydrates, or 65 percent fats, 30 percent protein, and 5 percent carbohydrates.

CYCLIC KETOGENIC DIET (CKD)

Designed for extreme athletes and bodybuilders, the cyclic ketogenic diet is typically five days of SKD followed by two carbohydrate-loading days. These are days when you intentionally eat a high percentage of carbohydrates. While there can be some variation of how many days to carb-load, the premise is to replenish the glycogen stores that can be lost during working out or bodybuilding.

TARGETED KETOGENIC DIET (TKD)

This is another approach used by athletes, in this case with the aim of using targeted carbohydrates to optimize their workouts. You would consume your entire carbohydrate allotment for the day 30 minutes before a workout, opting for fast-digesting carbohydrates like pure maple syrup. I'll cover exactly how I recommend to tweak and personalize your carbohydrate amount later on in the book.

RESTRICTED KETOGENIC DIET

With the constant availability of food most people have at their fingertips, it's uncommon for one to have ever given their body true fasting periods. A restricted ketogenic approach is used for those with chronic illnesses such as cancer or seizure disorders. The restriction comes from intermittent fasting and very low carbohydrate intake.

By having your body produce ketones and driving down glucose production, you are in effect starving many kinds of cancer cells and driving down inflammation. We'll look more at intermittent fasting in Chapter 7.

the health benefits of keto diets

It's easy to be skeptical or dismiss ketogenic diets as another food fad. After all, we are a society that is obsessed with the next, best thing. (We have truly seen it all, haven't we?) But this "diet," when done properly, is not about dieting at all, and it is based in biochemistry, not buzz alone.

The benefits of this approach to eating go far beyond just losing weight (even though that can definitely be one of the perks!). While each person has unique biochemistry that will manifest the positive results of keto differently and to varying degrees, most everyone experiences key benefits across the board.

MITOCHONDRIAL FUNCTION

Your body needs some sort of fuel in order to produce energy. Most people are used to all the carbs with big plates of pasta or munching on granola bars to get that boost. No one will argue that sugar doesn't give you a quick boost, but it will also leave you crashing later.

Ketosis takes us back to our cellular DNA roots—back to what our natural state is supposed to be. As babies, we rely on fat in the form of breast milk for energy and development, with no refined or grain sugar in sight. We begin life in ketosis and slowly move away from it, influenced by our culture's highly processed, sugary offerings.[8]

Mitochondria are the powerhouses of your body's cells. Their main responsibility is cellular respiration—that is, they take in nutrients, such as glucose, and break them down to turn into energy.

Adenosine triphosphate (ATP) is a molecule used by your cells for energy, and it is produced by metabolizing food. One unit of sugar produces thirty-six ATP molecules, whereas one unit of fat produces forty-eight ATP molecules. In short, fat provides us with more energy than sugar. In fact, a ketogenic diet has been shown to increase mitochondria biogenesis, or the making of new mitochondria.[9]

Who remembers the ice bucket challenge? The viral phenomenon originally started to support research for amyotrophic lateral sclerosis, also known as ALS or Lou Gehrig's disease. People with ALS tend to have reduced mitochondrial activity, which has shown promise of improvement through a ketogenic diet.[10]

REDUCED INFLAMMATION

Ketones like beta-hydroxybutyrate are not just a form of fuel—they're also a signaling molecule and epigenetic modulator, forging and supporting anti-inflammatory pathways. Chronic systemic inflammation is the underlying thorn in the side of almost all health problems. When you dive deeper into various illnesses, they tend to have one thing in common: inflammation. Anxiety, depression, fatigue, heart disease, and autoimmune conditions, all seemingly unrelated health problems, have their roots in inflammation.

To be clear, inflammation is not inherently bad. When you catch a virus or get a cut, acute inflammation is there to help repair damaged tissue and help fight off the intruder. But chronic inflammation over time, like a forest burning in perpetuity, fuels health problems. Remember that Goldilocks principle I mentioned earlier? That applies to inflammation as well. Too little and your body can't defend itself. Too much and your body is attacking itself, as we see with autoimmune conditions.

Today, there are close to one hundred recognized autoimmune diseases, with an additional forty that have an autoimmune component. There is no doubt that this number will continue to rise as science discovers autoimmune components to more diseases. Sadly, this is the age of autoimmunity. But just because something is ubiquitous doesn't make it normal—or mean that we can't do something about it.

It is estimated that just in America alone, fifty million people have been diagnosed with an autoimmune disease.[11] In most cases, the official diagnostic criterion is that the patient's immune system has already destroyed a significant amount of their body. For instance, a 90 percent destruction of the adrenal glands is required for a diagnosis of autoimmune adrenal issues or Addison's disease.[12] There also has to be major destruction of the neurological and digestive systems to be diagnosed with neurological autoimmunity like multiple sclerosis (MS) or gut autoimmunity such as celiac disease.

But this amount of autoimmune-inflammation attack did not happen overnight—it's the end stage of the larger autoimmune-inflammation spectrum. Overall, this process has three stages:

1. **Silent Autoimmunity:** There are positive antibody labs but no noticeable symptoms.

2. **Autoimmune Reactivity:** There are positive antibody labs and the patient is experiencing symptoms.

3. **Autoimmune Disease:** There's enough body destruction to be diagnosed and loads of potential symptoms.

In my functional-medicine center, I see many people in the second stage: not sick enough to be diagnosed, but nonetheless feeling the effects of autoimmune reactivity. People living somewhere on the inflammation spectrum often go from doctor to doctor, with a pile of labs and medications yet nothing to show for it. These patients are often essentially told, "Well, you will probably get lupus in a few years—come back then."

But what sense does it make to wait until you are unhealthy enough to be labeled with a disease to do something about it? Especially when at that point, for many, the only options typically given are steroids or immune-suppressing drugs. We can do so much better, and functional medicine, which treats the body using the healing power of nutrition, is leading the way.

The ketogenic diet does wonders for controlling other mechanisms responsible for chronic inflammation. For example, the Nrf-2 pathway regulates antioxidant gene induction and works to turn on genes responsible for antioxidant and detox pathways in addition to cell function and inflammation. When the Nrf-2 pathway is functioning at optimal levels, inflammation is calmed. When levels are low, inflammation is raised. The ketones produced in nutritional ketosis upregulate the Nrf-2 pathway and the powerful anti-inflammatory cytokine IL-10 and downregulate pro-inflammatory cytokines.[13]

When you are in a ketogenic state, the ketones your body produces and uses for fuel are powerful inflammation-fighting superheroes. Beta-hydroxybutyrate (BHB) works on inflammation by inhibiting the NLRP3 inflammasome—an inflammatory protein that is triggered by infections, tissue damage, or metabolic imbalances—which activates inflammation and has been implicated in a wide range of autoimmune-inflammatory diseases.[14]

Additionally, BHB activates the uber-important AMPK pathway involved in regulating energy balance and is able to reduce inflammation through inhibiting inflammatory

NF-kB pathways in the body.[15] BHB also has a similar effect on pain and inflammation as the nonsteroidal anti-inflammatory drug ibuprofen by inhibiting the COX-2 enzyme.[16]

There are actually two forms of this enzyme, COX-1 and COX-2. Ibuprofen blocks both of these enzymes, but COX-2 really causes our inflammation problems. COX-1, on the other hand, is found in your gut lining. That's why ibuprofen has been correlated with higher instances of leaky gut syndrome. Ketosis gives you the benefit of this medication without the negative impact to your digestive system and liver.

FLIPPING YOUR SELF-CLEANING SWITCH

Another benefit of the keto diet is that ketosis increases autophagy.[17] Literally translating as "self-eating," autophagy is your body's natural cleaning and recycling system. During autophagy, your healthy cells hunt down diseased and dysfunctional cells. Your healthy cells then eat the damaged cells and recycle them for energy and repair.

Autophagy is another way to make your cells stronger and more efficient, and a ketogenic state and intermittent fasting (more on that later) are two of the best ways to increase autophagy. Keeping autophagy at a healthy, active level is another way to keep your inflammation levels balanced and prevent accelerated aging and disease. Sounds good to me.

NEUROLOGICAL IMPROVEMENTS

Around 25 percent of your body's cholesterol is found in your brain,[18] and remember, your brain is composed of 60 percent fat.[19] Think about that. Over half of your brain is fat! What we have been traditionally taught when it comes to "low-fat is best" ends up depriving your brain of the very thing it is made of. It's not a coincidence that many of the potential side effects associated with statins—cholesterol-lowering drugs—are brain problems and memory loss.[20]

Your gut and brain actually form from the same fetal tissue in the womb and continue their special bond throughout your entire life through the gut-brain axis and the vagus nerve. Ninety-five percent of your happy neurotransmitter serotonin is produced and stored in your gut, so you can't argue that your gut doesn't influ-

measuring inflammation

If you are interested in getting your inflammation levels checked, these are the best labs to request:

- **CRP:** C-reactive protein is an inflammatory protein. It is also a surrogate lab to measure IL-6, another pro-inflammatory protein. They are both linked to chronic inflammatory health problems. The optimal range is under 1 mg/L.

- **Homocysteine:** This inflammatory amino acid is linked to heart disease and destruction of the blood-brain barrier and dementia; it is also commonly seen with people struggling with autoimmune issues. The optimal range is less than 7 Umol/L.

- **Microbiome labs:** Your microbiome is the term for the trillions of bacteria and yeast in our gut, in our mouth, and on our skin. We look to assess gut microbiome health, where around 80 percent of our immune system resides and a source for many people's chronic inflammation.

- **Intestinal permeability lab:** This blood test looks for antibodies against the proteins that govern your gut lining (occludin and zonulin), as well as bacterial toxins that can cause inflammation throughout the body, called lipopolysaccharides (LPSs).

- **Multiple autoimmune reactivity labs:** This array shows us if your immune system is creating antibodies against many different parts of the body, such as the brain, thyroid, gut, and adrenal glands. The labs are not meant to diagnose an autoimmune disease but to look for possible evidence of abnormal autoimmune-inflammation activity.

- **Cross-reactivity labs:** These tests are helpful for people who are gluten-sensitive and who have gone gluten-free and eat a clean diet but still experience digestive problems, fatigue, and neurological symptoms. In these cases, relatively healthy food proteins—such as gluten-free grains, eggs, dairy, chocolate, coffee, soy, and potatoes—may be mistaken by the immune system as gluten, triggering inflammation. To such a person's immune system, it's as if they have never gone gluten-free.

- **Methylation labs:** Methylation is the big biochemical superhighway that makes a healthy immune system, brain, hormones, and gut. It happens about a billion times every second in your body, so if methylation isn't working well, you aren't either. Methylation gene mutations, such as MTHFR, are highly associated with autoimmune inflammation. For example, I have a double mutation at the MTHFR C677t gene, which means that my body is not good at bringing down a source of inflammation called homocysteine. I also have autoimmune conditions on both sides of my family. By knowing my gene weaknesses, I can pay extra attention to supporting my body and lowering my risk factors as much as possible. For example, I have to be on point with eating green vegetables and sulfur-rich vegetables like cabbage and broccoli sprouts, which support healthy methylation pathways. I also have to be intentional with supplementing with methylated B vitamins.

Exciting emerging science is showing that a ketogenic diet can be more powerful than some of the strongest medications for brain-related problems.

ence the health of your brain.[21] The gut is known as the "second brain" in the medical literature, and a whole area of research known as the cytokine model of cognitive function is dedicated to examining how chronic inflammation and poor gut health can directly influence brain health.[22]

Chronic inflammation leads to not only increased gut permeability but blood-brain barrier destruction as well. When this protection is compromised, your immune system ends up working in overdrive, leading to brain inflammation.[23] Inflammation can decrease the firing rate of neurons in the frontal lobe of the brain in people with depression.[24] Because of this, antidepressants can be ineffective since they aren't addressing the problem. And this same inflammatory oxidative stress in the hypothalamic cells of the brain is one potential factor of brain fog.[25]

Exciting emerging science is showing that a ketogenic diet can be more powerful than some of the strongest medications for brain-related problems such as autism, attention deficit/hyperactivity disorder (ADHD), bipolar disorder, schizophrenia, anxiety, and depression.[26] Through a ketogenic diet, we can not only calm brain-gut inflammation but also improve the gut microbiome.[27]

Ketones are also extremely beneficial because they can cross the blood-brain barrier and provide powerful fuel to your brain, providing mental clarity and improved mood. Their ability to cross the blood-brain barrier paired with their natural anti-inflammatory qualities provides incredible healing properties when it comes to improving traumatic brain injury (TBI) as well as neurodegenerative diseases.[28]

Medium-chain triglycerides (MCTs), found in coconuts (a healthy fat option in the Ketotarian diet), increase beta-hydroxybutyrate and are proven to enhance memory function in people with Alzheimer's disease[29] as well as protect against neurodegeneration in people with Parkinson's disease.[30] Diets rich in polyunsaturated fats, wild-caught fish specifically, are associated with a 60 percent decrease in

Alzheimer's disease.[31] Another study of people with Parkinson's disease also found that the severity of their condition improved 43 percent after just one month of eating a ketogenic diet.[32] Studies have also shown that a ketogenic diet improves autism symptoms.[33] Contrast that with high-carb diets, which have been shown to *increase* the risk of Alzheimer's disease and other neurodegenerative conditions.[34]

TBI or traumatic brain injury is another neurological area that can be helped through a ketogenic diet. When a person sustains a TBI, it can result in impaired glucose metabolism and inflammation, both of which are stabilized through a healthy high-fat ketogenic diet.[35]

Ketosis also increases the brain-derived-neurotrophic factor (BDNF), which protects existing neurons and encourages the growth of new neurons—another neurological benefit.[36]

In its earliest phases, modern ketogenic diet research was focused on treating epilepsy.[37] Children with epilepsy who ate this way were more alert, were more well behaved, and had more enhanced cognitive function than those who were treated with medication.[38] This is due to increased mitochondrial function, reduced oxidative stress, and increased gamma-aminobutyric acid (GABA) levels, which in turn helps reduce seizures. These mechanisms can also provide benefits for people with brain fog, anxiety, and depression.[39]

METABOLIC HEALTH

Burning ketones rather than glucose helps maintain balanced blood sugar levels, making the ketogenic way of eating particularly beneficial for people with metabolic disorders, diabetes, and weight-loss resistance.

Insulin resistance, the negative hormonal shift in metabolism that we mentioned earlier, is at the core of blood sugar problems and ends up wreaking havoc on the body, eventually leading to heart disease, weight gain, and diabetes. As we have seen, healthy fats are a stronger form of energy than glucose. The ketogenic diet lowers insulin levels and reduces inflammation as well as improving insulin receptor site sensitivity, which helps the body function the way it was designed. Early trial reports have shown that type 2 diabetes symptoms can be reversed in just ten weeks on the ketogenic diet! [40]

Fascinating research has been done correlating blood sugar levels and Alzheimer's disease. In fact, so much so that the condition is now being referred to by some experts as *type 3 diabetes*. With higher blood sugar and increased insulin resistance comes more degeneration in the hippocampus, your brain's memory center.[41] It's because of this that people with type 1 and 2 diabetes have a higher risk of developing Alzheimer's disease. This is another reason to get blood sugar levels balanced and have our brain burn ketones instead.

If you are interested in assessing your own blood sugar, these are the labs that I run for my patients around the world:

- **Serum insulin (optimal range: <3 ulU/mL)**
- **C-peptide (optimal range: 0.8 to 3.1 ng/mL)**
- **Fasting blood sugar (optimal Range: 70 to 90 mg/dL)**
- **Hgb A1C (optimal Range: <5.3 percent)**
- **Triglycerides (optimal Range <100 mg/dL)**
- **HDL (optimal Range: 59 to 100 mg/dL)**

TAMING HUNGER AND ACHIEVING WEIGHT LOSS

Weight loss is a big reason why people first consider a ketogenic diet, and it's not until they've started their keto journey that they discover the other amazing benefits of this way of eating. But keto's amazing weight-management power can't be denied.

Multiple studies have shown that the ketogenic diet produces fewer feelings of hunger,[42] with dieters maintaining a much better mood than they do on other diets.[43] When's the last time you heard of being *happy* to be on a diet? And of course, that positive mood means you're more likely to stick with it.[44]

HEART HEALTH

We also can't fail to mention the elephant in the ketogenic room: heart disease. Eating this much fat can't possibly be good for you, right?! Well, I beg to differ. By lowering triglycerides and small dense, oxidized LDL, a high healthy-fat diet can actually *lower* your risk for heart disease by decreasing arterial plaque caused by a buildup of lipoproteins.[45] Have you already had a heart attack? A ketogenic diet has been shown to help with continued recovery.[46]

CANCER FIGHTING AND PREVENTION

Sadly, the American Cancer Society estimates that in one year alone just over 1.5 million people will be diagnosed with cancer.[47] Our DNA has stayed the same for thousands of years and has not caught up with the dramatic change in the food we eat and our environment, which are triggering our latent genetic predispositions like never before.

Many cancer cells heavily rely on glucose for their growth and metabolism, known as the Warburg effect.[48] Multiple studies have shown that the ketogenic diet can aid in reducing tumor size and growth of various cancers such as stomach,[49] lung,[50] and prostate cancer.[51] Even with severe brain cancer tumors like astrocytoma[52] and central nervous system tumors like glioblastoma multiforme,[53] a ketogenic diet has been shown to reduce tumor growth.

One major pathway that the ketogenic diet activates is the AMPK pathway, which can suppress the growth of tumors and its ability to inhibit a protein (mTOR) that's responsible for accelerated cell growth and division. Multiple studies have been done to show the correlation between the management of the mTOR pathway and the reduction of tumors in various cancers.[54]

MANAGING PCOS

Polycystic ovary syndrome (PCOS) is a metabolic disease that is correlated with abnormal glucose and androgen metabolism. This hormonal issue affects close to 10 percent of all women and causes many problems such as weight-loss resistance and fertility issues.[55] A ketogenic diet can help manage insulin sensitivity and therefore is a good natural treatment for this disease.[56]

potential problems with the ketogenic diet

The ketogenic diet has caught a lot of attention for its neurological improvements, weight-loss success, blood sugar regulation, and other compelling benefits. But there are also some potential pitfalls to eating this way over the long haul.

MACRONUTRIENTS OVER QUALITY

Just because a particular food is technically "keto" doesn't mean it's healthy or benefiting your body in any way.

Many great food products on the market are labeled as "keto friendly." I know of some awesome products such as pure avocado oil that are marketed specifically for the keto community. The problem we run into most often, however, is the additional treats and packaged products that are far from beneficial.

Where the ketogenic diet is concerned, it's easy to get so hyperfocused on macronutrients that we aren't conscious of the quality of the foods we're eating. As long as it fits into our macronutrient calculations for the day, many keto eaters will embrace it.

This leaves us consuming these problematic inflammatory foods such as conventional dairy and meat as well as artificial sweeteners that can harm our gut and put us on a path to chronic inflammation and health problems, despite our best intentions.

TOO MUCH DAIRY

In the average ketogenic diet, dairy is a major component, but is it helping us achieve optimal health? You probably grew up thinking milk was good for you. It has protein and calcium and because so many of us associate milk with childhood nutrition, it just seems like it is a healthy food. After all, it does a body good, right? However, for many people and for many reasons, dairy is inflammatory. Along with gluten, dairy is potentially one of the most inflammatory foods in our current diet, as well as being one of the most common food allergens.[57] Inflammation from dairy allergens or lactose intolerance affects millions of individuals, leading to symptoms that include gas, bloating, diarrhea, acne, joint pain, constipation, and eczema.[58]

Casein, the protein found in dairy, is the major culprit. Beta-casein, the main type, has two subtypes: A1 and A2. In the regular milk that you find in the grocery store, the A1 subtype is more common, because most cows in the United States have casein gene mutations due to thousands of years of crossbreeding. Unfortunately, A1 beta-casein is a trigger for digestive problems and inflammation.

And if that's not bad enough, most cows raised here are given hormones and antibiotics, live in unhealthy conditions, and are fed corn instead of grass, what they have grazed on for millennia. Their milk is then pasteurized and homogenized and the fat is removed. To make up for it having little nutrition, synthetic vitamins are then injected into the milk, trying to simulate what nature had already included in the whole-food form.

The problem with most dairy today isn't the dairy itself; it's what we have done to the cow. It's no wonder that dairy is causing so many issues in our population—and with dairy being a major component in the standard ketogenic diet, it is amplifying the damage.

For this reason, I suggest using ghee or clarified butter in the Ketotarian plan. Clarifying grass-fed butter removes the casein protein, leaving you only with grass-fed dairy fat, which is typically better tolerated.

AVOIDING PLANT FOODS

A common misunderstanding among many who follow the ketogenic diet is that vegetables are to be significantly limited. Since keto is a low-carb diet and vegetables contain varying amounts of carbohydrates, I have seen countless well-intentioned keto eaters grow fearful of consuming vegetables. Sadly, they are unwittingly missing out on the phytonutrients and prebiotic foods needed for a healthy gut microbiome.

Diets high in fats and low in plant fiber have been shown to drive up inflammation in the body.[59] A state of inflammation called metabolic endotoxemia begins with the gram-negative bacteria residing in the microbiome. These bacteria contain lipopolysaccharides (LPS), or bacterial endotoxins, in their cell wall. When LPSs enter the bloodstream because of intestinal permeability or leaky gut syndrome, they increase inflammation throughout the body. On the other hand, high-fiber diets like Ketotarian feed our beneficial bacteria, which produce beneficial metabolites and help lower inflammation.[60]

Another related problem with the ketogenic diet can be a loss of electrolytes, sodium, magnesium, calcium, and potassium, due to the natural loss of fluid retention. While sodium can be easily gained through seasoning foods with sea salt, potassium is a little harder to gain without eating plants—and it's important for cellular function as well as heart, brain, and kidney health.

The most common and abundant sources of potassium include the following:

- **Avocado:** 1,067 mg per 1 whole avocado

- **Spinach:** 839 mg per 1 cup spinach

- **Sweet potatoes:** 855 mg per 1 large potato

- **Kale:** 329 mg per ½ cup kale

- **Squash:** 896 per 1 cup squash

Magnesium is another vital nutrient that your body needs to thrive. In fact, it is the fourth most abundant mineral in your body and is needed for more than three hundred important biochemical reactions in your body.[61] There are many reasons why a person might be deficient in magnesium, such as gut problems and soil depletion, but poor dietary choices are at the top of the list.

It is estimated that between 50 and 90 percent of the population is deficient in magnesium. Lack of this mineral can lead to brain problems such as brain fog,[62] migraines,[63] anxiety, and depression[64] and can contribute to thyroid problems, since magnesium is necessary to produce thyroid hormones.[65] Since every cell of your body needs thyroid hormones to function, you can see the long-standing issue that can come from a lack of magnesium.

Just like potassium, the highest levels of magnesium can be found through plant foods such as the following:

- **Spinach:** 157 mg per 1 cup of spinach

- **Swiss chard:** 154 mg per 1 cup of chard

- **Avocado:** 58 mg per 1 medium avocado

PROCESSED AND CONVENTIONAL MEATS

Bacon lovers rejoice! On the conventional keto diet, lean meats are out of the question and all types of fatty cuts of meat are optimal as long as they come from high-quality sources.

Without a proper understanding of what's in your food, it can be tempting to go hog-wild on meat sources. After all, few diets advocate fats and meat consumption quite like the conventional ketogenic diet. But eating non-organic, grain-fed conventional meats is a source of inflammation and is widely linked to cancer and other health problems.

For many potential reasons, processed meats like lunch meats and many bacon, jerky, and sausage products are linked to cancer and other diseases. Eating conventionally raised and processed meats is doing nothing for your health, even if it's "low-carb, high-fat."[66]

Some people, depending on their genetics or gut health, do better with less of even the organic meats in their diet. This is another reason I created Ketotarian—for those who want to get in on all the next-level health benefits of ketosis but don't do well eating (or don't prefer) more red meat.

As we'll see, there's a way to enjoy the benefits of keto principles without these pitfalls. But first, let's look at the standard plant-based diet as it's commonly followed.

2 | plant-based diets
(For Better and Worse)

When you think of a healthy diet, one of the first images that probably comes to mind are baskets filled with fresh fruits and vegetables. In the wellness world, vegetarian and vegan diets are often used as the poster children for the ultimate clean eating.

In fact, the rate of people choosing to eat a vegan diet, without any meat or dairy, has gone up a whopping 500 percent from 2014 to 2017. Now, 6 percent of Americans identify as vegan compared to just 1 percent a few years ago. It's not just veganism that has increased—becoming more plant-based in general is increasing in popularity. For example, in 2017, 44 percent of Germans followed a low-meat diet, which is significantly higher than the 26 percent in 2014.

The growing awareness of the benefits of plant food sources is undeniable. Science shows us repeatedly how eating a diet rich in vegetables help reduce disease risk and health problems. An estimated $1 trillion in yearly health care costs and lost productivity would be saved if we went more plant-based—not to mention the benefit it could have on the health of our environment.[1]

benefits of plant-based eating

DETOXIFICATION

As a society, we are surrounded by more toxins than ever before. On a daily basis, we are exposed to dubious chemicals in the products we use and genetically modified foods sprayed with pesticides and herbicides in our grocery stores and restaurants. Our genetics have not caught up with this onslaught of toxins, and it is evident in the rise of inflammation-spectrum health problems.

Even with our best efforts for living a clean, green life, it is virtually impossible to avoid all toxins. Plus, the question isn't just how much we are exposed to toxins, but also what our body's individual genetic tolerance to them is.

> The last thing we need is another quick-fix detox. Instead, we need to make our lives a cleanse—and plants are just what your body ordered.

Some people can handle many stressors in life, including toxins, while others can't. Someone might smoke three packs of cigarettes a day and live to be eighty while the next person could die from secondhand smoke at forty. It doesn't mean smoking is healthy—but it does show that we all have different thresholds for toxins.

Many people, including me, have methylation impairments such as the MTHFR methylation gene mutation. Not only do these gene changes increase your chances of autoimmunity, but they also inhibit your body's ability to remove toxins from your system.

Toxins are another piece of the autoimmune puzzle. As I have mentioned before, autoimmune conditions are just the end stage of the larger autoimmune-inflammation spectrum, and toxins are just another contributor to chronic inflammation.

Toxins surround us every day, even in the places that we don't always think twice about. However, some common toxins are implicated in the initiation, progression, and exacerbation of autoimmune disease:[2]

- **Mercury:** found in some seafood and amalgam teeth fillings

- **Vinyl chloride:** found in some tap water, vehicle upholstery, and plastic kitchenware

- **BPA:** found in many common plastic products

- **Heavy metals:** found in some tap water as well as many skin, hair, and cleaning products

- **Organic solvents:** found in some paints, varnishes, lacquers, adhesives, glues, and cleaning agents, and in the production of dyes, plastics, textiles, printing inks, agricultural products, and pharmaceuticals

- **Formaldehyde:** found in many skin, shampoo, and cleaning products

- **Pesticides:** found in nonorganic foods and water supply

And ladies, if you frequently dye your hair, you are potentially exposed to toxins like p-phenylenediamine, formaldehyde, resorcinol, and more, all of which have been implicated in cancer and hormone dysfunction.[3]

The last thing we need is another quick-fix detox. Instead, we need to make our lives a cleanse—and plants are just what your body ordered. Plants have developed powerful detoxification mechanisms of their own. Certain antioxidant phytonutrients, phytochelatins, and metallothioneins are considered heavy-metal binders that help to protect plants from the effects of these toxins, and by consuming these plant sources they can protect you as well.[4] One study found a dramatic increase in metallothioneins (a powerful detoxifier) production in women who increased their consumption of phytonutrient-dense foods, such as the green leafy vegetable watercress.[5]

Some of the most powerful phytochelatin antioxidants are sea vegetables like chlorella and spirulina and herbs such as parsley and cilantro (as if you need another reason to indulge in a cilantro-topped taco bowl! Pass some of that healthy-fat-loaded guacamole as well!).

Onions, broccoli, broccoli sprouts, Brussels sprouts, cabbage, cauliflower, and mushrooms all support methylation detox pathways. By bringing these foods into your diet on a regular basis, you are supporting detox and naturally making your life a cleanse.

Folate, another essential vitamin needed for healthy methylation pathways, can be found in dark leafy greens like kale, collards, spinach, and chard.

REDUCED INFLAMMATION

Plant medicines are great at calming inflammation levels. Increasing polyphenols like metallothionein also inhibits inflammatory NF-kB signaling, which has been implicated in the pathogenesis of many chronic inflammatory conditions.[6] At the same time, polyphenols found in plant-based sources such as vegetables, fruit, spices, and herbs also bring down NF-kB and activate anti-inflammatory Nrf-2.[7] Some of my favorites include the following:

- **Green tea**

- **Blueberries**

- **Ginger**

- **Curcumin (found in turmeric)**

Plant foods also increase your peroxisome proliferator-activated receptors (PPARs), which may help improve inflammatory conditions such as heart disease, asthma, colitis, MS, and other autoimmune conditions. PPAR activators include green tea, ginger, sea buckthorn, astragalus, and loads of vegetables. (By the way, ketosis and wild-caught salmon also improve PPARs.)

Do you remember our friend Nrf-2, the protein that plays a role[8] in regulating antioxidant function? The Nrf-2 pathway actually turns on genes that are responsible for antioxidant and detox pathways. Inflammation is calmed when Nrf-2 is activated, and it is worse when there are low levels of Nrf-2.

Many dietary antioxidants have been found to activate Nrf-2, including the following:

- **EGCG from green tea**

- **curcumin from turmeric**

- **rosmarinic acid from rosemary**

- **L-sulforaphane from broccoli**

- **thiosulfonate allicin from garlic**

ENHANCED MICROBIOME HEALTH

Plants are food for your microbiome, allowing your gut bugs to make short-chain fatty acids (SCFAs). SCFAs are produced in your body when good gut bacteria ferments fiber in your colon. Where does your gut get this fiber? Largely from plant foods.

One of the main SCFAs in your body is butyrate, which has powerful anti-inflammatory effects on the gut. Butyrate boosts the health of your digestive and immune system and improves irritable bowel syndrome (IBS), ulcerative colitis, and Crohn's disease.[9]

REDUCED ASTHMA

In a study of processed red meat consumption and asthma symptoms, eating cured meat four times a week increased the likelihood of asthma flares by a staggering 76 percent.[10]

LOWER BLOOD SUGAR

Another benefit of going plant-based can be improved blood sugar levels and reduced risk of diabetes. Many studies have shown that people who consume a pre-dominantly plant-based diet have dramatically lower rates of diabetes.[11] In a long-term study of over two thousand men followed over nineteen years, replacing even 1 percent of calories from animal proteins with plant proteins lowered the risk of developing diabetes by 18 percent.[12]

CANCER FIGHTING AND PREVENTION

Multiple studies have shown that eating either a vegetarian or vegan diet significantly lowers your cancer risk. Research from many studies points to a connection between an increase in colon cancer rates and eating processed red meat[13]—and it doesn't stop with colon cancer. When looking at the research, you can see the wide-sweeping conclusion that plant-based diets are the best choice when it comes to reducing your chances for being diagnosed with many kinds of cancer.[14]

All of these studies showing the various health benefits of a ketogenic diet and plant diets are impressive, but remember that correlation does not necessarily mean causation. Some of these studies do not have randomized control trials, which is considered the gold standard in the health research world. While more studies are, of course, always welcome, plenty of strong evidence shows the beneficial applications of both the ketogenic and plant-based diets.

We can also put the research aside for a moment and use real life as a lab (novel idea, right?). Research is important, but sometimes we overvalue being "evidence-based" over common sense and self-experimentation—paying attention to what works in your life and what doesn't, what improves your health and what doesn't. That's evidence too. For every study in the medical literature showing that something delivers health benefits, there is a dissenting opinion or study. I could write a book about how grass is green and I would probably hear a rebuttal.

So test the tools in this book for yourself. Give it a real, concerted effort. Don't worry, I'll walk you through everything you need.

IMPROVED ENVIRONMENT

This benefit of going plant-based isn't a direct health benefit, but it is paramount for our health and sustainability as a society, long term. Shifting our diet to being richer in plants can make a major impact the environment, the health of the earth we live on. If cattle were their own nation, they would be the world's third-largest emitter of greenhouse gases.[15]

> Shifting our diet to being richer in plants can make a major impact on the environment and the health of the earth we live on.

Plant-rich diets reduce emissions and also tend to be healthier, leading to lower rates of chronic disease. Emissions could be reduced by as much as 70 percent through adopting a vegan diet and 63 percent for a vegetarian diet.[16] If 50 percent of the world ate about 2,500 calories a day and lowered their meat consumption, it is estimated that at least 26.7 gigatons (that's 26 billion tons!) of emissions could be avoided from diet change alone. If the avoided deforestation from land use change is factored in, an additional 39.3 billion tons (gigatons) of emissions could be avoided! This makes healthy, plant-rich diets one of the best solutions for making a positive impact on our environment.[17]

With that said there are many wise voices that say sustainable cattle farming can, in fact, reduce global warming. People like Joel Salatin and Allan Savory point out that two-thirds of the earth's grasslands are turning to desert. One hundred sixteen miles of soil is exported daily and 75 billion tons every year by conventional farming. Moving cattle to mimic wild grazing animals, they say, will heal the man-made damage to our environment. This waste is more than twenty times the amount of food needed for every living person on the planet. Sustainable, holistic farming will allow cattle to churn and fertilize the soil. This symbiotic relationship helps to promote healthy microbes and carbon into the soil instead of the atmosphere.[18]

There is no doubt that environmental solutions are a nuanced issue. No one will argue, though, that it would do our planet a great service to eat plenty of plants and for those of us who choose to eat meat, we should do so from organic and sustainable sources.

Before we jump into this best-of-both-worlds plant-based ketogenic plan, let's go over some of the potential pitfalls of the typical plant-based diet.

where plant-based diets go wrong

Vegetarian and vegan diets done wrong can lack nutrients and fuel inflammation. Let's take a closer look to avoid these common plant-based pitfalls.

CARBATARIANS AND INFLAMMATARIANS

The average vegan or vegetarian often fills up with carbohydrates and packaged processed food. Sadly, the food industry has taken the plant out of the plant-based diet.

Many vegans and vegetarians have been led to believe that "healthy" whole-grain carbs are what we need for sustainable energy. This belief causes one of the biggest problems with a conventional plant-based diet.

When done correctly, a plant-based diet can provide you with the nutrients needed to thrive. However, too often grains become the staple of the modern plant-based diet.

We live in a grain-centric society; grains are the foundation of what people buy in the grocery stores. The next time you are grocery shopping, just take a look at what's in the other carts. Grains are the foundation of what most people have on their plates: cereal for breakfast, a sandwich for lunch, and a grain as a side (at least) for dinner. They're the backbone of industrial farming, which is a multibillion-dollar juggernaut in politics and policy. Grains are even the foundation of the infamous food pyramid (or a huge slice of the USDA MyPlate), which educates the general public on what we should be eating.

It's no surprise, then, that even the idea of eliminating grains sounds radical to many. People can get defensive and protective about their grains. The addiction runs deep.

But a report in the *American Journal of Clinical Nutrition* explains how we've seen a rapid change in our world over a relatively short period of time.[19] Our current food supply, soil depletion, and environmental toxins have all been new introductions to human existence. Put another way, around 99 percent of our genes were formed before the development of agriculture and the consumption of grains like wheat, around ten thousand years ago.

> Around 99 percent of our genes were formed before the development of agriculture and the consumption of grains like wheat, around ten thousand years ago.

Researchers now argue that these factors are essentially a mismatch with our genes. And more recent refining, hybridization, spraying, and genetic modification of the grain supply have likely only made things worse. Our genes are living in a whole new world.

Bottom line: grains (and a lot of other foods) are not what they once were. And in our modern, toxic world, we have less wiggle room for unhealthy foods than generations before us did. It's just a matter of someone's own genetic interaction with grain, especially gluten-containing grains, that determines if, when, and how a health problem will be triggered.

When we consume high amounts of grains we quickly start to raise our blood sugar, which over time can get out of control without us even realizing it. Grains are also high in sugars. These grain sugars overwhelm your body, causing insulin spikes and a hormonal hurricane of insulin resistance, high triglycerides, and inflammation—hallmarks of chronic disease.

Grains are also high in a class of sugars called FODMAPs. This funny-sounding acronym stands for *fermentable oligosaccharides, disaccharides, monosaccharides, and polyols*—in other words, fermentable sugars. These short-chain sugars are not fully digested in your gut and can be excessively fermented by your gut bacteria. This fermentation releases hydrogen gas that causes distension of the intestines—which can cause major IBS and small intestinal bacterial overgrowth (SIBO), with symptoms like pain, gas, bloating, constipation, and diarrhea.

GLUTEN SENSITIVITIES

With grains, though, it's not just about the sugars like the FODMAPs, it's also about the proteins. Researchers estimate that around eighteen million Americans have a "gluten sensitivity." The growing awareness of gluten, the protein found in grains such as wheat, rye, barley, and spelt, has spawned an endless vortex of gluten-free everything. Gluten-free desserts, gluten-free crackers; you probably could even find gluten-free gluten if you searched hard enough!

What's the bottom line? Is gluten something you should avoid, or is it an overblown fad reminiscent of the "fat-free" movement that had little to no health merit? Is gluten intolerance actually real?

One trial published in *Clinical Gastroenterology and Hepatology* studied people who thought gluten was causing them digestive problems.[20] The gold standard for research is a randomized, double-blind, placebo-controlled, crossover trial, and gluten was put to this rigorous test—and this study checked all the boxes. For one week participants were given either a small amount of gluten or a placebo pill of rice starch. After only one week, those who were taking the gluten pills reported a significant increase in symptoms compared to those who took gluten-free placebo pills. Other randomized control trials have shared similar findings.[21]

To understand gluten intolerance, we need to understand autoimmune conditions. Many people think when we talk about gluten intolerance we are referring to the autoimmune condition celiac disease. Celiac disease is really the extreme end of a broader gluten-intolerance spectrum. The other end of that spectrum is nonceliac gluten sensitivity (NCGS).

What are the symptoms of gluten intolerance?

People in the study noticed the following:

- **Abdominal bloating**

- **Ulcers**

- **Intestinal pain**

Because your gut is your "second brain," people with gluten intolerance can also experience the following:

- **Brain fog**

- **Depression**

- **Anxiety**

- **Fatigue**

What most people don't realize is that your body could be reacting to more than twenty different aspects of wheat. Most patients who ask to be tested for gluten intolerance get a simple alpha-gliadin lab test. If it comes back negative you are told you are not gluten intolerant. You may want to then celebrate the good news by eating a basket of breadsticks, but not so fast. Alpha-gliadin and the common celiac lab test for transglutaminase 2 are just two pieces of about a twenty-piece wheat puzzle.

LECTINS AND PHYTATES

Lectins are another type of protein found in grains, even the gluten-free ones like rice and corn. These grain defense mechanisms are highly indigestible by the body. When your gut is damaged by this mild toxin, your body's defense systems are compromised, causing inflammation.[22] Lectins can also bind to insulin and leptin receptor sites, causing hormonal resistance patterns such as weight-loss resistance.[23]

If you haven't already found yourself emptying your cupboards, then we can talk about phytates. Grains also contain these nutrient leeches. Phytates are antinutrients that bind to minerals in your body and make them unusable. The little nutrients that grains do offer are diminished by phytates, which make them unavailable for your body.[24] Therefore, it doesn't really matter how many nutrient-dense vegetables you are having if you end up counteracting their benefits.

Along with those guys, saponins are antinutrients that are high in pseudograins, like quinoa, which is a popular staple among many plant-based diets. Saponins can damage your gut, leading to increased gut permeability, which can contribute to inflammation and chronic conditions.

It's important to remember that grains today are not what they were in the past. With crossbreeding and genetic modification, grains are chemically different today than they were even a few decades ago. A common argument for eating grains is to get in an adequate amount of fiber. However, vegetables offer ample amounts of fiber (not to mention a whole slew of other nutrients) without the number of offenses to your gut, brain, immune system, and hormones.[25]

Another primary food in typical plant-based diet is legumes. This category encompasses all types of beans, lentils, and peanuts. Because of their protein content, they have become a typical stand-in for meat in many vegetarian and vegan lifestyles. The problem here is that lectins and phytates are also found in legumes in high amounts, similar to grains.

SOY

We cannot talk about legumes without talking about the ever-controversial soy. It is difficult to find a product, plant-based or not, that doesn't contain soy these days. And for vegans and vegetarians it's one of the most common ingredients in nonmeat products because of its high protein content.

Soy is considered a complete protein as well as a phytoestrogen. Soy is rich with plant-based estrogens, known as isoflavones, which your body does not produce through the endocrine system. Instead, they are gained through eating phytoestrogenclassified plants. Out of all phytoestrogens, soy is the most well known and has been praised for many years as a hormone replacer because of its isoflavone content. But phytoestrogens can affect your hormones in a big way, mainly for men and women who have issues with estrogen dominance, because they can block the more potent natural estrogens from binding to the estrogen receptor, leading to hormone imbalance.

But like grain, soy hasn't always been an issue like it is today. Fermented soy products such as natto and tempeh have been consumed by many healthful cultures for years. "Second-generation" soy products, however, incorporate chemical extractions using hexane and aluminum and other processing, and encompass soy protein isolate and soy flour. These products become the main ingredients in items such as meatless burgers, dietary protein supplements, and infant formula, and are also used as nonnutritive additives to processed foods.[26] Most of the soy that is consumed in our food industry is genetically modified. In fact, most of the soy produced in the United States is genetically modified.[27]

Plant-based dieters typically also enjoy nuts, such as almonds, cashews, and hazelnuts. Most people, however, aren't aware that proper preparation is key for actually getting the nutrients that nuts carry and avoiding any indigestion that may occur from mass-produced nuts and seeds that make their way onto grocery shelves. Studies indicate that phytate-mineral complexes are insoluble in the intestinal tract, reducing mineral bioavailability.[28] Phytates also have been shown to inhibit digestive enzymes such as trypsin, pepsin, alpha-amylase, and beta-glucosidase.

Therefore, ingestion of foods containing high amounts of phytates could theoretically cause mineral deficiencies or decreased protein and starch digestibility. Soaking our nuts, seeds, and legumes can drastically change the way we digest these health foods and allow us to actually reap the benefits that they are designed to give. It's like these foods are dormant or asleep, but by soaking them we awaken their properties and prepare them to deliver what we want. We take the time to clean our fruit and vegetables, so why not properly prepare our nuts, seeds, and legumes?[29]

NUTRIENT DEFICIENCIES

If you are filling your plate with more grains and legumes rather than fresh vegetables, you are probably going to run into some health problems sooner or later. But we can even see the lack of nutrients play out in many plant-based diets that don't rely heavily on those two food groups.

Many studies link vegetarian and vegan diets to deficiencies in key nutrients including vitamin D, magnesium, B vitamins, and iodine—all nutrients that if lacking can lead to hormonal, thyroid, and methylation impairments. Many of these nutrients are available only in animal sources, and the ones that are found in plant sources do not have the same level of bioavailability. And the sources that do have decent nutrient levels also contain phytates, which end up blocking nutrient absorption. For example, phytates bind to zinc and iron, which we will discuss in more detail later, resulting in low absorption of these in the body. So unfortunately, with a plant-based diet we can end up living off many foods that not only are inflammatory and cause digestive distress but also inhibit our body from making use of the vital nutrients we're consuming.[30]

For the most part, while vegetarian and vegan diets can both lead to major nutrient deficiencies, you typically see this less in vegetarians than in vegans because they usually still eat some type of animal product such as eggs. Either way, let's take a deeper look at the most common deficiencies and why plant-based diets don't always make the cut in this department.

DHA AND EPA

Omega fatty acid deficiencies in the standard vegan diet are the subject of a long-held argument. But if you are feeling better from not eating meat, is it that important to worry about not getting these omega fatty acids? A well-balanced diet with natural sources of alpha-linolenic acid (ALA) and the long-chain omega-3 fatty acids DHA and EPA is fundamental to maintaining a healthy ratio that prevents inflammation and promotes long-term health by protecting against health problems like autoimmune and cardiovascular disease. Additionally, your brain is composed of about 60 percent fat, so depriving your body of fat can contribute to all kinds of unpleasant brain symptoms, from brain fog and fatigue to depression and anxiety. In other words, healthy fat is essential for optimal brain health.

It is vital to consume these fatty acids because they can't be synthesized by the body, and diet is the only way to get them in. Before you argue that plant-based dieters can get these omega fats through plant-based sources such as legumes, nuts, and seeds, let's talk about how bioavailable these sources actually are.

The average American consumes a large amount of their omega-3s in the form of ALA. These are derived from plant sources. ALA is an energy source for our cells, and a small percentage of this is converted into DHA and EPA.[31] In fact, only up to 10 percent of EPA and up to 5 percent of DHA actually end up being converted in the body.[32] The amplest amounts are found in fatty, cold-water fish sources such as salmon, trout, cod liver, herring, mackerel, and sardines, and in shellfish such as shrimp, oysters, clams, and scallops. These sources of omega-3 are the most bioavailable to your body.[33] Vegetarians have an estimated 30 percent deficiency in both EPA and DHA; vegans have a 50 percent deficiency in EPA and a 60 percent deficiency in DHA.[34]

With ALA being a large source of our omega-3 consumption, and the only source for vegans, it is vital to consume DHA and EPA sources. And yes, that may mean incorporating some fish or at least algae like spirulina (which also contains bioavailable omegas) into your diet.

VITAMINS A AND D

Fat-soluble vitamins in particular are some of the worst deficiencies that we see in vegans and vegetarians. This is because these two vitamins are almost exclusively found in animal-based foods such as organ meats, eggs, dairy fats like ghee, and wild-caught seafood.

No other vitamin can hold a candle to vitamin D when it comes to importance and influence on health. Since vitamin D is fat-soluble, it acts more like a hormone than a vitamin by regulating thousands of vital pathways in your body. Besides your thyroid hormones, this vitamin is the only other thing every single cell of your body needs in order to function properly. Also known as the sunshine vitamin, vitamin D is synthesized by your body when your bare skin is exposed to sunlight. But it is impossible to get enough vitamin D from food alone, and unless you live in a very sunny place (closer to the equator) and if you are outside frequently without sunscreen or tons of clothing, you are probably deficient.

Since vitamin D deficiency is already a problem for most of the population, omnivores included, it is even greater for plant-based dieters. Typically, vegetarians and vegans, on average, have more vitamin D deficiencies compared to meat eaters.[35]

Vitamin A is essential for a strong immune system, and vitamin A deficiency has been linked to autoimmune diseases, which are on the rise in a major way.[36] Some researchers believe this has to do with our dendritic cells, which are our alarm cells of the immune system that can send out a "red alert" to stimulate immunity, or a "calm down" message that tones down excessive immune reactions that can damage the body. The "calm down" message uses vitamin A.

Plant beta-carotenes, a precursor to vitamin A, are found in sweet potatoes and carrots, but the conversion rate to the usable form of vitamin A, retinol, is very weak. In fact, research suggests that just 3 percent of beta-carotene gets converted in a healthy adult.[37] Because of this, you can see how deficiency can be common among people who eat a vegan or vegetarian diet. You'd have to eat a rather large amount of carrots and sweet potatoes to even attempt to reach adequate levels.

B_{12}

This is potentially the biggest deficiency for all types of plant-based diets. B_{12} is absolutely necessary for methylation, your body's biochemical superhighway that happens more than 1 billion times a second in your body to keep you alive and healthy. It is your DNA protection system; it controls how efficiently you detox, and every single cell of your body depends on this process. In short, if methylation is not working well, a lot can go wrong with your health.

True B_{12} is found only in animal products such as wild-caught fish, grass-fed beef, eggs, and dairy products. A common alternative of plant-based B_{12} often comes from sea vegetables like seaweed and spirulina, as well as fermented soy. However, these don't contain true B_{12}. Instead they are B_{12} analogs known as cobamides, which are not as bioavailable.[38]

For vegan and vegetarian dieters, this is one nutrient that no matter what or how much you choose to eat, you'll never truly be able to reach optimal levels without supplementation. In fact, it's estimated that 68 percent of vegetarians and 83 percent of vegans are deficient in this vital vitamin.[39]

And that's not taking into account any possible genetic weaknesses. A mutation in your MTR/MTRR methylation gene, which regulates B_{12} production, can require higher intakes of B_{12} than normal since the body ends up using B_{12} faster than it can produce it.

ZINC

Your body has no significant way to store this important mineral, so it's important to make sure you're getting it through your diet or supplementation. Zinc's main role is to help your body increase white blood cells and fight off infection, and it also assists with the release of antibodies. Deficiency has been linked to increased instances of illness,[40] so it's no wonder you often find zinc as a common ingredient in the cold and flu aisle of your pharmacy. It's especially important for pregnant women since it is required for proper fetal growth and development.[41]

This is a very easy nutrient to get through a plant-based diet. But what we often see is that typical plant foods that contain zinc still contain phytates, which block nutrient absorption. So if intake is not monitored, zinc deficiency can still happen and often requires more zinc-containing foods to reach necessary daily intake levels.

IRON

Iron is needed to get oxygen to your cells. And if your cells are deprived of oxygen they don't function properly and well, and not much else in your body does either. Some typical symptoms I see with low iron are fatigue and low sex drive.

There are two ways to look at iron levels in your body. One is serum iron, which measures the levels of iron currently circulating in your blood. The other is ferritin, which measures long-term iron storage in the body. The serum levels of most vegetarians and vegans are similar to those of meat eaters, but the difference is seen when it comes to ferritin levels.

While we definitely don't want ferritin levels to be too high, which is correlated with increased inflammation, we don't want them to be low either, which is a sign of iron deficiency.

There are also two different types of iron—heme and non-heme. Heme is the most bioavailable iron for your body and is found only in meat. Non-heme isn't absorbed as easily and is found in dairy, eggs, and plant foods.

Many plant foods contain iron, but only the non-heme variety. Dark leafy greens, mushrooms, nuts and seeds, and legumes all contain high amounts of iron, but if you are consuming too many legumes you'll run across problems with phytates decreasing your absorption. Additionally, iron absorption can be inhibited by other substances that are consumed such as calcium, coffee, and tea. And again, plant sources just do not have the same level of bioavailability as animal sources. All of these factors contribute to an 85 percent lower non-heme iron absorption rate in plant-based diets.[42]

As our deficiencies continue to escalate, so does our need to supplement. For vegans and vegetarians, all of these deficiencies can be mitigated through regimented supplementation—but if the foods we eat are missing some key bioavailable nutrients, are we on the right path? Maybe. Maybe not.

3

the new keto:
Plant-Based Ketogenic Alchemy

my journey from low-fat vegan to ketotarian

The evolution of my health journey started years ago when I was a student in college, when I first decided not to eat any animal products. It came from a well-intentioned place—I had educated myself on factory farming, concentrated animal feeding operations (CAFOs), where animals live in deplorable conditions, and the damage that eating animals causes our health and environment.

I thought I knew it all. I was going to tell anyone who would listen about how being a vegan was better than what they were doing.

Today, I see the tenacity of my youth for what it was, a form of egotistic superiority. Turning our noses up at people who don't feel the same way we do is an ugly look. Now I realize that we are all on our own journey and we should honor each other. That doesn't mean we can't share what we have learned, but we should do it respectfully and without judgment.

The turning point in my life was when I started studying functional medicine. I learned about getting to the root causes of illnesses and realized there's no "one size fits all" approach to wellness. I had to come to grips with the fact that I was eating healthfully but wasn't *feeling* healthy. Something was missing.

So, after ten years as your typical strict vegan, I quit—and now I feel better than ever.

Was veganism better for me than the standard American diet? Certainly! But for me, just because something was better didn't make it optimal. I hesitated even writing this book. In my years writing about functional-medicine health topics, I've received the most online vitriol from the vegan community. Those tactics don't change minds; they only divide.

From my own personal health journey, and now seeing thousands of patients both as a human being and as a functional-medicine practitioner, I came to the conclusion that pure veganism wasn't the answer for me. Here's why:

MY DIGESTION WAS WRECKED

I believe that years of not eating healthy, organic meat and fat contributed to hypo-chlorhydria, or low stomach acid, and gallbladder issues. (I found this out by running functional medicine labs on myself.) This made it difficult for my body to digest foods. That, along with all the grains and legumes I was eating, contributed to intestinal hyper-permeability or leaky gut syndrome.

MY DETOX PATHWAYS WERE WEAK

It's estimated that about 40 percent of us have methylation dysfunctions, such as MTHFR mutations, and I am one of them. Methylation is the biochemical superhighway that helps with your detoxification system, brain, gut, and immune health. This mutation could increase the risk of chronic brain, hormonal, digestive, and autoimmune conditions.

Choline and vitamins B_9 (folate) and B_{12} are essential for healthy methylation pathways—and these three nutrients are abundantly found in wild-caught fish. Sure, I could supplement, but if I can't get these nutrients naturally from the foods I'm eating, is my diet really optimal for my body?

MY SKIN WAS BREAKING OUT

My skin is very prone to acne breakouts. When I was vegan, in addition to my wrecked gut health, I also wasn't getting enough beneficial vitamin A from the foods I was eating—and both contributed to unhealthy skin.

Retinol, what's sometimes called true vitamin A, or the bioavailable form, is found only in animal products like fish, shellfish, egg yolks, cod liver oil, and grass-fed ghee. Plant carotenes, a precursor to vitamin A, are found in sweet potatoes and carrots—but, as I mentioned previously, the conversion rate to the usable retinol is poor.

Once I started optimizing my diet with true vitamin A-rich sources like cod liver oil, and foods rich in collagen (which also can't be gained naturally through plants) like wild-caught marine collagen, I noticed that my skin improved.

MY IMMUNE SYSTEM WAS WEAK

I often found myself run down. In addition to a lack of healthy fats, it was also due to a lack of fat-soluble vitamins. Vitamin A is essential for equipping you with a strong immune system. And vitamin A deficiency has also been linked to autoimmune diseases such as rheumatoid arthritis and type 1 diabetes.

Why? Dendritic cells, the alarms of the immune system, stimulate immunity, or calm down excessive immune inflammation that can damage the body. You need true vitamin A (retinol) to send this "calm down" message to your immune system.

Vitamin D is also essential for many metabolic and immunological pathways in the body. For example, Th17 cells are helper T cells that produce a number of inflammatory chemicals, such as interleukin-17. With autoimmune conditions—such as inflammatory bowel disease, multiple sclerosis, psoriasis, and rheumatoid arthritis—Th17 cells are out of control.

Vitamin D, in conjunction with vitamin A, has been shown to synergistically dampen the Th17 inflammatory response. As with vitamin A, vitamin D is most abundant in fish, egg yolks, and ghee. But soaking up some time in the sun can also help—about 20 to 60 minutes a day, depending on your complexion. And consider getting tests done every few months to ensure that your vitamin D levels are healthy.

In addition to vitamins A and D, there is also the often-overlooked fat-soluble vitamin K_2. One study in the *Journal of Neuroimmunology* found that vitamin K_2 was effective at inhibiting the pro-inflammatory iNOS in the spinal cord and the brain immune system in rats that had multiple sclerosis symptoms.[1] Unfortunately, K_2 is one of the most common nutrient deficiencies in the Western diet.

Vitamin K_2 is best paired with the other fat-soluble vitamins, A and D, in wholefood form like grass-fed butter oil (ghee). Natto, a Japanese superfood made from non-GMO fermented soybeans, also has high levels of K_2.

I HAD BRAIN FOG AND FATIGUE

I believe that a lack of healthy fats during my low-fat vegan diet contributed to the brain fog I experienced. After all, the omega fats found in fish are a superfood for the brain.

Sure, omega-3 fat ALA can be found in plant sources such as walnuts and flaxseeds, but as I mentioned earlier, it's not easily used by our bodies because it must be converted into DHA or EPA, which is an inefficient process.

My energy crashes went hand in hand with my fatigue. Arachidonic acid and docosahexaenoic acid are two forms of fat that could play an important role in brain health. And the most bioavailable sources for these brain foods? Fish and other animal sources. Iron was also another deficiency in my strict low-fat vegan diet, ample in clean seafood.

These days, we're struggling with an undeniable epidemic of inflammatory brain and neurological problems. Anxiety, brain fog, fatigue, depression, attention deficit disorder (ADD), autism, Alzheimer's disease, Parkinson's disease, and multiple sclerosis—the long list of conditions affects nearly everyone in some way.

And with more people than ever before battling these brain issues, we have to ask ourselves: why? While there are many complex reasons for the decline in society's health in the modern world, let's talk about what I feel is one of the main culprits.

For years, fat and cholesterol have been demonized in our diets. Since the latter part of the twentieth century, we've been told these nutrients would clog our arteries and cause us to gain weight, and we've avoided them.

Even today this belief remains—but its days are numbered. A study in the medical journal *Neurology* found that, contrary to popular belief, there might actually be no association between high total cholesterol and stroke risk.[2] In fact, other research has shown that low cholesterol may actually increase the likelihood of death. At the same time, some of the many side effects of statins—cholesterol-lowering drugs—include memory loss and brain dysfunction.[3]

As the fattiest organ in your body, your brain is composed of mostly fat, and a quarter of all your body's cholesterol is found in your brain. Consuming cholesterol and fat is critical to the health and function of the brain—but for years we've been starving our brain from its favorite food.

WHAT HAPPENED AFTER I WENT KETOTARIAN

So there I was, a staunch vegan with health problems creeping into my life. Was I going to continue not eating any animal products just so I wouldn't have to admit that

I was wrong? My dear friend and colleague Dr. Terry Wahls, who was a vegetarian for years herself, said poignantly:

> I spent some time reflecting on life in the wild. We all consume one another in the end. Our atoms and molecules are continually recycled. Every living thing without the benefit of photosynthesis must consume other beings—plants, fungi, bacteria, and animals. And in the end, they will consume me.
>
> I prayed and meditated on these ideas. Humans have been eating all these things for thousands of generations, so I decided I was not committing a crime against nature if I ate meat. Perhaps I was getting even closer to nature.

I also realized that I was not separate from or above nature but a part of it. And because of my MTHFR methylation impairments and digestive and skin issues—as well as a family history of autoimmune conditions—pure veganism was not right for my long-term health.

Now that I'm eating the plant-based, high-healthy fat ketogenic meals in this book, I feel better than ever—and so can you. My energy is great, and my skin and digestion have dramatically improved, all benefits you can enjoy too.

While Ketotarian is almost entirely plant-based and would be considered ketogenic-vegan, it also uses a few key food medicines to give more variety of healthy fats. Some of the Ketotarian recipes also include ketogenic-vegetarian options, bringing in foods such as the following:

- **Eggs:** Pasture-raised, organic egg yolks are rich in nutrients such as vitamins A, D, E, and B; choline; iron; calcium; phosphorus; and potassium, which all contribute to healthy hormones, brain, immune system, and skin.

- **Ghee:** Grass-fed ghee or clarified butter has had the often-inflammatory dairy protein casein removed, leaving the butterfat with its fat-soluble vitamins A, D, and K_2, all needed for a healthy immune system, brain, hormones, and skin. Ghee has a high smoke point, making it a good option to cook with.

I also am introducing another option in your Ketotarian food plan that would be considered ketogenic-pescatarian:

- **Wild-caught fish and shellfish:** By bringing in the world's healthiest wild-caught fish, you get bioavailable omega fats and minerals needed for optimal brain, hormone, immune, skin, and metabolic health. While some may call this pescatarian, we are avoiding carb-heavy legumes and grains like most pescatarian diets. Because we are focusing instead on all the delicious vegetables our world has to offer, we are more accurately vegaquarian!

Other than these three food medicines in some recipes, Ketotarian is entirely plant-centric. Although these three additions to a Ketotarian approach are ultimately optional, and you can go completely plant-based, I added these in for specific reasons that were born out of my own health journey and now the thousands of patients I have seen from around the world over the years.

ketotarian: the new age of ketosis

Whether you're a vegan or vegetarian, eat a conventional ketogenic diet or paleo diet, or eat whatever the heck you feel like, you can't look around and be OK with the decline of our collective health. With the rise of autoimmune conditions and other chronic health conditions, despite spending trillions of dollars, a change has to be made.

Food is more than just a meal, it's fuel and information for every organ, tissue, and cell in our body. This is why Ketotarian is the solution you've been looking for. We've seen where ketogenic and plant-based diets go right and where they fall short. Ketotarian is the ultimate hybrid of these two eating styles, designed to give your body every single thing it needs for optimal health.

Ketotarian is in complete alignment with human physiology and our DNA. This high-fat, nutrient-dense lifestyle stays true to the ketogenic ways and is as plant-based as you get, while remembering the importance of reducing inflammation, promoting healthy gut function, and intentionally using food medicines to heal the body.

Practically speaking, Ketotarianism is sustainable and user-friendly, because when you are fat-adapted you feel satisfied and don't experience cravings—a top reason that most diets fail. When you have switched your metabolism to bringing ketones, you are officially off the blood sugar roller coaster, resulting in food freedom at last.

I created the Ketotarian plan for the vegan, vegetarian, ketogenic, and standard American (or Western culture as a whole for that matter) eater alike who wants to optimize their health. Whether you never want to eat meat or just want to add more plant-based ketogenic ideas into your life, this is your home. Today, I eat with grace and lightness. Most of my life is plant-based, but if I want to have wild-caught fish one day or even grass-fed beef another, I will.

By using the tools in this book, I shifted my body to fat-adaptation. As a lifestyle, I now have the metabolic flexibility to increase healthy carbs when I feel like it, then go back to nutritional ketosis as my metabolic foundation.

I eat intuitively now, in tune with what my body truly needs. Ketotarianism transcends dogma, beyond shame and dieting rules and fine print. This is the new age of eating.

> Ketotarianism transcends dogma, beyond shame and dieting rules and fine print. This is the new age of eating.

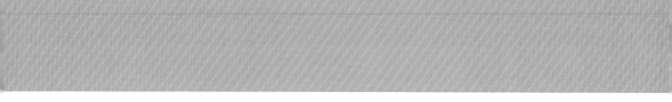

4 | ketotarian foods:
What to Eat and What to Avoid

Welcome to Ketotarian Land. This is where we dig into all the delicious, nutrient-dense, filling foods you get to eat on your plant-centric ketogenic plan. Forget survival—this is your thrival guide.

Remember:

60-75 percent of your calories should come from fat (but it can be more!)

15-30 percent of your calories from protein

5-15 percent of your calories from carbohydrates

In the beginning of your Ketotarian journey, as the body is becoming fat-adapted, most people do best by eating somewhere between 25 and 55 grams of net carbs daily. Net carbs are just total carbs minus fiber and sugar alcohols like xylitol. For most people, fiber and sugar alcohols don't affect blood sugar levels or get stored as glycogen.

what to eat

HEALTHY FATS

Fat is your fuel. Focusing on healthy fats and cutting unhealthy carbs to curb cravings is the secret to becoming fat-adapted. This will make you a fat-burning, anti-inflammatory, anti-aging, brain-fueling powerhouse. Have some fat at every meal. Depending on your size and amount of activity, your fat intake should be about 20 to 60 grams per meal.

So, what kinds of fats should you be eating? It's a nuanced issue, because you can actually turn good fats into bad fats with improper cooking. Many people pick a great fat but unintentionally turn it into a bad one by overcooking beyond the smoke point and oxidizing the fat, causing inflammation in the body. Using extra virgin olive oil to fry foods is a good example of this. It's important to know the smoke points of the oils you are using, which is why I have divided the good-fat list into those appropriate for cooking and those that should be eaten unheated. But here's the takeaway: good fat is good for you, so don't skimp. Start off slow and work your way back up to the level of fat the human body is meant to consume and what works best for you.

FOR COOKING:

- Coconut oil
- Grass-fed ghee (clarified butter)
- Avocado oil
- Olive oil (other than extra virgin or virgin, which are for room temperature use)
- Hazelnut oil
- Macadamia nut oil
- Palm fruit oil
- Palm kernel oil
- Dark roasted sesame oil (lower temperature stir-fries)

FOR EATING WITH/ON/IN FOOD:

- Extra virgin olive oil
- Extra virgin coconut oil
- Avocado oil
- Walnut oil
- Flaxseed oil
- Hazelnut oil
- Almond oil
- Macadamia nut oil
- Hemp seed oil
- MCT oil
- Palm kernel oil
- Cocoa butter
- Grass-fed ghee (clarified butter)
- Avocados
- Guacamole
- Full-fat coconut milk
- Coconut meat
- Coconut cream
- Unsweetened coconut milk yogurt
- Unsweetened almond milk yogurt

A word on fats: There are some people who, because of different SNPs (genetic changes) such as the APOE4 allele or underlying gut problems, do better with moderating their saturated fat intake. In Ketotarian land that would mainly be coconut oil and ghee. For these people, focusing too much on saturated fats can increase inflammation. If you find that you don't do well (increased inflammation levels on labs or you just don't feel as good) on higher amounts of saturated fats, try limiting saturated fat intake to 30 grams/day. Focus instead on monounsaturated fats (olive oil, nuts, and seeds) and omega polyunsaturated fats.

NUTS AND SEEDS

Nuts are great sources of both fat and protein. Enjoy them solo, on salads, blended in smoothies, used to make nut milks and cheeses, or as grain-free flour alternatives.

- **Almonds** (6 grams protein + 14 grams fat per 23 nuts)

- **Brazil nuts** (4 grams protein + 19 grams fat per 6 nuts)

- **Cashews** (4 grams protein + 13 grams fat per 18 nuts)

how to soak nuts and seeds

Activate your nuts! Break up those inflammatory lectins and phytates with these simple steps.

1. **In a bowl, pour water over the nuts or seeds that you want to soak.**

2. **Add 1 to 2 tablespoons of your favorite sea salt.**

3. **Cover the bowl and let them soak on the counter or in the fridge for about 7 hours, or overnight.**

4. **Rinse the nuts or seeds to remove the salt and spread them out on a rack to dehydrate.**

5. **Dry the nuts or seeds in a dehydrator until they are slightly crispy. If you don't have a dehydrator, you can roast them in your oven at a low temperature until they are slightly crispy. If you choose not to dry them, they typically will last in the fridge for a few days before they can become moldy.**

If soaking nuts and seeds isn't your thing, there are brands that sell soaked and sprouted nuts and seeds.

- **Chia seeds** (4 grams protein + 9 grams fat per 2 tablespoons)

- **Flaxseeds** (4 grams protein + 8 grams fat per 2 tablespoons)

- **Hazelnuts** (4 grams protein + 17 grams fat per 21 nuts)

- **Hemp seeds** (11 grams protein + 13.5 grams fat per 3 tablespoons)

- **Macadamia nuts** (2 grams protein + 22 grams fat per 11 nuts)

- **Pecans** (3 grams protein + 20 grams fat per 19 nut halves)

- **Pine nuts** (4 grams protein + 20 grams fat per 165 nuts)

- **Pistachios** (4 grams protein + 18 grams fat per 49 nuts)

- **Sacha inchi seeds** (9 grams protein + 16 grams fat in 40 seeds)

- **Walnuts** (4 grams protein + 18 grams fat per 14 nut halves)

A word on nuts and seeds: the roughage of nuts and seeds (more so with nuts, less with seeds), as well as the protein lectins and phytates, can irritate some people. Plus most nuts sold in stores are typically coated in inflammatory industrial seed oils, like soybean or canola oil. They could also contain partially hydrogenated trans fats, which can contribute to problems as well. Make sure you are going for raw nuts and seeds and properly preparing them. I find that most people do better with soaking nuts and seeds in water overnight to break down the inflammatory lectins and make their nutrients more bioavailable.

PASTURE-RAISED EGGS

This incredible, edible superfood is one of the most unjustly and inaccurately perse-cuted foods ever. The yolk of the egg gets a particularly bad rap, despite containing most of the egg's nutrients. I see so many well-intentioned people throw out the yolk or buy egg whites out of misplaced concerns about fat and cholesterol. In fact, the egg yolk is truly nature's multivitamin.

6 grams protein + 5 grams fat per egg (3 to 4 eggs would give you around 20 grams of fat!)

what does this amount of fat look like per meal?

You are probably thinking this sounds like a heck of a lot of healthy fats. You may be surprised. The average person can begin to aim for around 30 grams of fat for every meal as they are starting out. What does that look like?

Food	Amount	Fat content	Amount per meal
Almonds	10 nuts	6 grams	20 to 30 almonds
Almond butter	1 tablespoon	10 grams	3 tablespoons
Avocado	1 whole	30 grams	1 avocado
Coconut cream	1 tablespoon	5 grams	6 tablespoons
Coconut oil	1 tablespoon	14 grams	2 tablespoons
Eggs	1 egg	5 grams	3 to 4 eggs
Ghee	1 tablespoon	15 grams	2 tablespoons
Macadamia nuts	10 nuts	21 grams	15 nuts
Olive oil	1 tablespoon	14 grams	2 tablespoons
Pecans	10 nuts	20 grams	15 nuts

Organic, pastured eggs from chickens who roam outside in the sunlight offer us essential brain food like choline and omega-3 fats. As with all meat and dairy, not all eggs are created equal. Pasture-raised eggs have been shown to contain *three times* more of the brain-beneficial omega-3 fats than supermarket eggs.

A final word on eggs: I find that the egg white is potentially more inflammatory for some people. The protein in the white, albumin, could pass through the intestinal lining if you have leaky gut syndrome, contributing to inflammation. If you don't tolerate eggs, consider duck eggs. They are also typically better tolerated than chicken eggs.

PLANT PROTEIN

Remember, your Ketotarian plan is high fat, low carbohydrate, and moderate protein. Aim for around 0.5 to 1 gram of protein per pound of lean body weight every day. Your lean body weight or mass (LBM) is the amount of weight on your body that isn't fat. There are many calculators online that easily allow you to calculate your LBM. The average optimal protein intake range for a person with 100 pounds of lean body mass would come to 45 to 68 grams per day. In addition to nuts and eggs, here are some plant protein options to bring into your day.

- **Hempeh (tempeh made from hemp seeds):** 22 grams protein per 4 ounces hempeh

- **Natto (organic non-GMO):** 31 grams protein per 1 cup natto

- **Tempeh (organic non-GMO):** 31 grams protein per 1 cup tempeh

- **Hemp protein powder:** 12 grams protein per 4 tablespoons powder

- **Hemp hearts/seeds:** 40 grams protein per 1 cup hemp

- **Maca powder:** 3 grams protein per 1 tablespoon maca

- **Peas:** 9 grams protein per 1 cup cooked peas

- **Nutritional yeast:** 5 grams protein per 1 tablespoon yeast

- **Sacha inchi seed protein powder:** 24 grams protein per 4 tablespoons powder

- **Spirulina:** 4 grams protein per 1 tablespoon spirulina

- **Almond butter:** 6 grams protein per ¼ cup butter

- **Spinach:** 3 grams protein per ½ cup cooked spinach

- **Avocado:** 2 grams protein per ½ avocado

- **Broccoli:** 2 grams protein per ½ cup cooked broccoli

- **Brussels sprouts:** 2 grams protein per ½ cup sprouts

- **Artichokes:** 4 grams protein per ½ cup artichokes

- **Asparagus:** 2.9 grams protein per cup asparagus

PRODUCE

This is the *tarian* of Ketotarian. While your average ketogenic diet can lead people to shun vegetables because of their carb content, the Ketotarian knows all the benefits of plant foods:

- **Disease-fighting phytonutrients**

- **Detox support**

- **Gut-health microbiome fuel**

Dark leafy greens like kale, spinach, and chard contain folate, which is essential for methylation and opening up detox pathways. Bitter greens like collard greens, mustard greens, and arugula are also great at supporting liver function. Broccoli sprouts contain the chemical compound glucoraphanin, which turns to sulforaphane in the body to aid in detoxification. Plants like parsley and cilantro work to eliminate heavy metals such as lead and mercury. Other sulfur-rich vegetables such as garlic, onions, Brussels sprouts, cabbage, and cauliflower help with methylation and liver clearing. All of these plant-food medicines offer fiber, which is food for your gut microbiome—all the trillions of bacteria that make up the majority of your immune system.

Please buy organic vegetables whenever possible. If you don't buy organic, be sure to wash your produce well. Fill the sink with cold water and add 1 cup white vinegar. Allow the fruits and vegetables to soak for 15 minutes. Rinse, pat dry, and store. For more information on the most pesticide-tainted vegetables and those that are less contaminated and okay to buy non-organic, see the list of the Dirty Dozen and Clean Fifteen published and updated yearly by the Environmental Working Group.

Vegetables

I recommend eating 4 to 9 cups per day of these nonstarchy to lower-starch vegetables. Aim for having at least 1 cup of vegetables with every meal at the start, then work up from there depending on your size, appetite, and sensitivity to carbs. Fill your plate with a variety of nutrient-dense vegetables for the optimal Ketotarian meals.

- Alfalfa sprouts
- Artichokes
- Arugula
- Asparagus
- Bean sprouts
- Beets
- Bok choy
- Broccoli
- Broccoli sprouts
- Brussels sprouts
- Cabbage
- Carrots
- Cauliflower
- Celery
- Chard
- Chives
- Collard greens
- Cucumber
- Dulse
- Endive
- Ginger
- Jicama
- Kale
- Kelp
- Kohlrabi
- Kombu
- Leeks
- Lettuce
- Mushrooms
- Nori
- Okra
- Olives
- Radishes
- Rhubarb
- Rutabaga
- Scallions
- Seaweed
- Spinach
- Swiss chard
- Turnips
- Water chestnuts

SPICES

Enjoy fresh or dried in any amount, to taste.

- Allspice
- Anise seed
- Annatto
- Caraway
- Cardamom
- Celery seed
- Cinnamon
- Clove
- Coriander
- Cumin
- Fennel
- Fenugreek
- Garlic
- Ginger
- Horseradish
- Juniper
- Juniper berry
- Mace
- Mustard
- Nutmeg
- Peppercorns
- Poppy seed
- Sea salt
- Sesame seed
- Star anise
- Sumac
- Turmeric
- Vanilla bean (no additives)

HERBS

Enjoy fresh or dried in any amount, to taste.

- Basil
- Bay leaf
- Cilantro

- Dill
- Lavender
- Lemon balm

- Mint
- Oregano
- Parsley

- Rosemary
- Sage

BEVERAGES

- Water

- Coffee (should be organic)

- Tea (should be organic)

- Coconut/almond milk (unsweetened)

- Kombucha (look out for too much added sugar; the more tart, the better)

- Carbonated water (no added sweeteners)

- Green juices (fresh-pressed green vegetables, lemon, lime, and ginger only; be mindful of the sugar content)

- Organic bone broth: One exception in the vegan/vegetarian/vegaquarian rules of the Ketotarian plan is bone broth made from organic chicken bones. Loaded with minerals and electrolytes, this nutrient-dense, gut-soothing food is something I suggest bringing into your Ketotarian lifestyle. With that said, you can always try fish broth, which would be vegaquarian compliant. But since fish broth isn't so mainstream, and not many people's cup of broth, organic chicken bone broth can be a great option.

KETOTARIAN BAKING

We are going beyond "gluten-free" here. Here are your *grain-free* options for baking.

Flour	Fat	Protein	Net carbs
Almond flour (¼ cup)	14 grams	6 grams	3 grams
Coconut flour (2 tablespoons)	3 grams	2 grams	2 grams
Chia seed meal (2 ounces)	17 grams	8 grams	3 grams
Flaxseed meal (2 tablespoons)	18 grams	3 grams	1 gram
Shredded Coconut (3 tablespoons)	10 grams	1 gram	2 grams
Tigernut flour (¼ cup)	7 grams	2 grams	9 grams

These numbers (and macronutrients in general) will vary depending on the brand or food-tracking calculator you are using.

You can also use xanthan gum instead of cornstarch for baking.

LOWER-FRUCTOSE FRUITS

We are limiting fruit sugars, so depending on your tolerance to sugar, have up to 2 small handfuls per day. Lemons, limes, grapefruits, and berries are the best choices as they are the lowest in fruit sugar.

- Blackberries
- Blueberries
- Cantaloupe
- Clementine
- Grapefruit
- Honeydew melon
- Kiwi
- Muskmelon
- Oranges
- Papayas
- Passion fruit
- Pineapple
- Raspberries
- Rhubarb
- Strawberries
- Tangelos

LOW-CARB NATURAL SWEETENERS

Use in small amounts to sweeten things up, to taste.

- Erythritol
- Inulin
- Monk fruit
- Stevia
- Tagatose
- Xylitol

net carbohydrates or total carbohydrates

OK, we are about to get super science nerdy. But I'll break it down and make it easy(ish) to understand. Basically, total carbohydrates are all carbs found in your food; net carbohydrates, on the other hand, are total carbohydrates minus the fiber and sugar alcohols. For example:

Food	Total Carbs. (g.)	Fiber (g.)	Sugar (g.)	Net Carbs. (g.)
1 Avocado	17.1	13.5	1.3	3.6

Carbs from real foods like vegetables and avocados contain both insoluble and soluble fiber. Insoluble fiber such as cellulose and lignin can't be absorbed by the body and has no effect on blood sugar and ketosis.

On the other hand, soluble fiber such as galacto-oligosaccharides and fructooligosaccharides (FOSs) are fermented by the gut microbiome into beneficial end products of bacterial fermentation called short-chain fatty acids (SCFAs): acetate, propionate, and butyrate. The concern in the mainstream ketogenic world is that soluble fiber can increase blood sugar levels, therefore negatively impacting ketosis.

But studies have shown that soluble fiber can actually lower blood sugar levels.[1] How, you ask? Well, the SCFA propionate is used by the body for intestinal gluconeogenesis (IGN), making glucose in the intestines. Through the IGN pathway, SCFAs actually bring about a net decrease in blood sugar. So, unlike liver (hepatic) gluconeogenesis, IGN seems to have a blood sugar balancing effect on the body. The beneficial ketone beta-hydroxybutyrate has similar benefits and structure as the SCFA butyrate produced from the resistant starch of plant foods.

In addition to all this science stuff, fiber can help with curbing cravings: ketosis + fiber from real food = craving-crushing magic. Win-win.

Ketotarianism focuses on nutrient-dense, real foods like vegetables, nuts, and seeds, which all contain carbs that are buffered and harnessed by whole-food fiber. In short:

1. **When you are eating nonstarchy vegetables, avocados, low-fructose fruits, and nuts and seeds on the Ketotarian plan, count net carbs.**

2. **If you eat processed, boxed foods (even the healthy ones) or any foods other than a real whole food, don't fool yourself: count total carbohydrates.**

As you are starting out on your healthy ketogenic path, most people do best around 25 grams net carbs (with a max of 55 grams net carbs) per day all from nonstarchy veggies and whole foods such as nuts and seeds. Since we are all different, I'll cover carb tweaking in more detail a little later.

NIGHTSHADES

Limit these, or avoid them altogether if you have autoimmune-inflammation issues. This plant group contains alkaloids in their skin that can cause an inflammatory response in the body to varying degrees depending on your health and sensitivity.

- Eggplant
- Goji berries
- Peppers (bell peppers, chili peppers, paprika, tamales, tomatillos, pimentos, cayenne)
- Potatoes (other than sweet potatoes)
- Tomatillos
- Tomatoes

KETOTARIAN / VEGAQUARIAN

OK, so now that we have gone over all the Ketotarian foods that would be considered vegan or vegetarian, let's talk about another special aspect of the Ketotarian kingdom.

We live on a planet covered by majestic deep blue seas. In fact, 70 percent of the earth's surface is underwater. Our climate and health are both intimately connected to the ocean, as half the oxygen we breathe is being produced by plants growing in the sea. It makes sense that if the sea is our source of life here on earth, then the ocean could contain secrets to our health that just don't exist on land. Let's explore exactly how to tap into the power of the sea to expand our health.

Fish such as wild-caught salmon, sardines, rainbow trout, Atlantic mackerel, and shellfish like mussels and oysters are rated by the Environmental Working Group as the best fish for you and the environment for their high amounts of omega-3 fats, low mercury levels, and sustainability factors. The ones you want to avoid because they have higher levels of toxins are larger predatory fish such as marlin, orange roughy, shark, swordfish, and tilefish.

We need omega fats. Many Americans have a 12:1

> Our climate and health are both intimately connected to the ocean, as half the oxygen we breathe is being produced by plants growing in the sea.

and up to a 25:1 ratio of omega-6 to omega-3 in their bodies, and ideally you want a 1:1 ratio to stay balanced. Omega-3 deficiency comes with unhealthy skin, poor sleep, and brain fog. Omega-3s are also needed to make your brain's neurotransmitters, with low levels of omega fats being linked to depression and anxiety. Wild-caught fish have these brain-, hormone-, heart-, and immune-supporting omega fats. The great thing about these clean fish, though, is that they are in whole-food form, not a supplement or powder. This allows the presence of variety of different nutrients, minerals, and fats that can't be encapsulated in a pill or a scoop.

But can't you get omega fats from nuts and seeds like chia and flax? Yes, but the problem is bioavailability, meaning your body's ability to access and use them.

Remember, there are two different forms of omega-3:

- **A short-chain plant-based omega-3 called ALA found in chia, flax, hemp, and walnuts**

- **Long-chain omega-3 fatty acids called EPA and DHA, found in fish, omega-3-rich eggs (chickens that are fed flax convert short-chain omega-3s into long-chain omega-3s for humans), and algae like spirulina**

All the anti-inflammatory benefits seen in the medical literature are from long-chain EPA and DHA omega-3, not ALA.

Studies indicate that the conversion of ALA to EPA and DHA is extremely limited. Less than 5 percent of ALA gets converted to EPA, and less than 1 percent of ALA is converted to DHA. Obviously enjoying nuts and seeds is still a great part of the Ketotarian plan, but in terms of meeting omega requirements it's just not efficient or the same.

If you are a plant-based vegan you should be taking an algae-based omega-3. If you are vegetarian, choose omega-3-rich eggs. And if you want to become a Ketotarian-vegaquarian, my favorite source is wild-caught fatty fish.

There are so many ways to enjoy fish, so have whatever floats your boat here. I love fish tacos and use lettuce wraps for a grain-free twist.

If you have not been eating meat and have decided to try reintroducing it, start off bringing meat in slowly to wake up your GI system. Many people who have eaten a vegetarian or vegan diet have low stomach acid, making it difficult to digest protein.

You may want to consider taking a digestive enzyme and betaine HCL supplements with pepsin to help your digestion out in the beginning, until your body adjusts.

Unless you are allergic to fish or shellfish, seafood is an excellent source of nutrition. These are the low-mercury seafood items I recommend. You can now officially call yourself a vegaquarian.

If you are going to eat these healthy seafoods, aim for about 1 to 2 palm sizes per meal and focus on the fattier varieties (** = highest amount of omegas, * = a decent amount of omegas)

- Alaskan salmon, wild-caught**
- Albacore tuna (U.S./Canada, wild, pole caught)**
- Anchovies**
- Arctic char
- Atlantic mackerel**
- Barramundi
- Bass (saltwater, striped, black)
- Butterfish
- Catfish*
- Clam
- Cod (Alaskan)*
- Crab (domestic)
- Croaker (Atlantic)
- Flounder*
- Herring**
- Lobster*
- Mahi mahi (U.S./Ecuador, pole caught)
- Mussels*
- Oyster**
- Pacific halibut*
- Pollock
- Rainbow trout**
- Rockfish*
- Sardines**
- Scallops
- Shrimp*
- Skipjack tuna (U.S./Canada, wild, pole caught)
- Sole (Pacific)*
- Squid (calamari)
- Tilapia
- Tuna (canned, chunk light)
- Whitefish
- Yellowfin tuna (U.S. Atlantic, wild, pole caught)*
- Yellowfin tuna (Western Central Pacific, wild, hand/line caught)*

ketotarianisms

—

1. Eat real food.

2. Keep your carbs low.

3. Keep your healthy fats high.

4. If you eat a nonstarchy vegetable, add some healthy fats.

5. If you eat a healthy fat, add some nonstarchy vegetables.

6. Eat when you are hungry.

7. Eat until you are satisfied.

—

the ketotarian triangle

LOW-FRUCTOSE FRUITS
*berries • lemons
limes • grapefruit*

LOW-STARCH VEGETABLES
*onions • broccoli
Brussels sprouts • cabbage*

CLEAN PROTEIN + GREENS
nuts • seeds • tempeh • fish • leafy greens

HEALTHY FAT
*coconut oil • coconut cream • avocados
avocado oil • ghee • olive oil • olives • eggs*

what not to eat

Ketotarianism is not about shame or using food to punish your body—it's about going for foods that fill you up, reduce inflammation, make you a fat-burner, and leave you feeling freaking fantastic. Let's reframe the way we look at food. This isn't about focusing on all the foods we "can't" have. You ultimately *can* eat whatever you want in life. These are just the foods that increase inflammation, raise your blood sugar, take you out of ketosis, or aren't healthy enough for you. Love your body enough to nourish it with good food medicine. Eating healthy foods is a form of self-respect. So, after you read this list, go back and focus on all the foods you get to enjoy instead.

SUGAR

Any added sugar. Anything with the suffix *–ose*. Read food labels, because sugar comes in a lot of fancy-sounding names.

Artificial Sweeteners

Just because these are "low-carb" doesn't mean they are healthy. (More on this later in the chapter.)

- **Sucralose**—Splenda

- **Aspartame**—Equal, NutraSweet

- **Saccharin**—Sweet'N Low

- **Neotame**—a chemical derivative of aspartame found in various food products

- **Acesulfame**

BAD FATS

Bad fats include trans fats like partially hydrogenated fats and highly refined poly-unsaturated industrial seed oils like canola, vegetable, and soybean oil, which are highly inflammatory.

DAIRY

Other than grass-fed ghee (clarified butter), avoid dairy in the Ketotarian plan.

GRAINS

That's all grains, my friend. Wheat, oat, rice, corn (yes, it's a grain, not a vegetable), rye, spelt, barley, buckwheat, and quinoa. Any product made from these grains such as bread, pasta, cereal, cakes, pastries, and beer should also be avoided.

HIGH-FRUCTOSE FRUIT

Other than the sweet guys on the lower-fructose fruit list, avoid fruit during your time in ketosis.

STARCHY VEGETABLES

Starchy vegetables include sweet potatoes (any potatoes, for that matter), yams, and plantains. Some starchy vegetables are used in the carb moderating tools later in the book, to further personalize your Ketotarian lifestyle.

A word on fruit and starchy vegetables: After at least 60 days of focusing and enjoying the keto-friendly foods and allowing the body time to become fat-adapted, some people do fine eating more fruit and starchy veggies. I will talk more about personalizing your Ketotarian lifestyle long term.

LEGUMES

Legumes include lentils, black beans, pinto beans, white beans, peanuts, soybeans, garbanzo beans, fava beans, kidney beans . . . all the beans.

Podlike legumes like peas and green beans and fermented non-GMO soy (natto and tempeh) are typically better tolerated and are allowed on your Ketotarian plan.

After 60 days, if you want to bring some legumes back in, give it a try—but note that their carb count can throw some people out of ketosis more easily than other foods.

A word on legumes: When eating legumes, I suggest soaking them for at least

8 hours before drying or cooking and eating them. Cooking beans and other legumes such as lentils in a pressure cooker is also an option. Soaking or using a pressure cooker will drastically reduce the potentially inflammatory lectin and phytic acid content of these foods.

MEAT

Other than the option of lower-mercury, wild-caught fish, we are eliminating meat. After 60 days if you want to bring in grass-fed beef or organic chicken a few times a week, this can be an option for you. Your diet will still be predominantly plant-based.

ALCOHOL

You may lose some friends (or gain some if they need a designated driver), but alcohol is doing pretty much nothing for you. We want the liver to be super healthy, and consuming alcohol can put an added stress on your liver—not what you want when shifting from being a sugar-burner to a fat-burner. I recommend trying at least 60 days without alcohol at the beginning of your Ketotarian journey. If you want to bring back some alcohol in small amounts later on, the best way is straight up with no extra sugars and syrups. Organic dry red wine is a decent option.

decoding sweeteners: the good, the bad, and the ugly

Wherever you look in the grocery store or restaurants, sugar is added to just about everything—it's in nut butter, condiments, kombucha, crackers, popcorn, and most everything else that comes in a package. This sweet drug of choice comes by many names, even healthy-sounding euphemisms, so it can be hard even recognizing sugar in all its varying forms.

I will tell you exactly which ones to avoid and the ones that are the recreational drugs of the sugar family: to be used responsibly, with caution, and in small amounts.

THE UGLY
Artificial Sweeteners

These chemical sweeteners actually can change the bacterial balance of your microbiome.[2] This can be a trigger for autoimmune problems, diabetes, and metabolic disorders. The following are the most common culprits, whose colorful packages you often see at any coffee bar:

- **Sucralose**—Splenda

- **Aspartame**—Equal, NutraSweet

- **Saccharin**—Sweet'N Low

- **Neotame**—a chemical derivative of aspartame found in various food products

- **Acesulfame**—often found in sodas and fruit juices as well as dairy and ice cream products

High-fructose corn syrup

This sweetener is so widely used that it can be shocking to learn just how many products actually contain it, even foods that you wouldn't think would contain any sweetener. It is derived from stalks of corn through an intensive chemical process that is anything but natural. Because of its chemical makeup, it does not need to be digested by your body and quickly enters your bloodstream, leading to insulin spikes that contribute to hormonal problems like leptin resistance, which increases weight gain and weight-loss resistance.

THE BAD
Agave Nectar

Because agave nectar is low on the glycemic index, a way of measuring how fast certain carbohydrates will raise your blood sugar, it is often touted as a healthier alternative. In my opinion, this is an overly simplistic way of determining whether a food is "bad" because you aren't considering any other factors. Agave nectar is still high in fructose, which can delay damage to the body. Although it is a slower process, your body still converts fructose into glucose, glycogen, lactate, and fat in your liver. This places stress on your liver and can contribute to insulin resistance and fatty liver disease.

Turbinado

Also known as raw cane sugar, this type of sugar is not so "raw" and unrefined. It still undergoes processing, which removes some of its natural impurities as well as nutrients. While it's still far less processed than refined white sugar, it's still not much better for you.

Brown Rice Syrup

This sweetener is made from a combination of brown rice and enzymes. The enzymes break down the starch, and then it is boiled down to create a syrup. The fermentation makes the sugars easier to digest. The big issue, though, is that barley enzymes are often used, which contain gluten. Unless you are specifically looking for gluten-free brown rice syrup, you could be unknowingly perpetuating health problems if you are sensitive to gluten.

Arsenic can start to build up in large amounts of rice. Studies have shown that arsenic levels have been found to be high in organic brown rice syrup used in a wide range of products. Make sure to limit your packaged products in which this sweetener is used to decrease toxin exposure.

THE DECENT BUT NOT KETOTARIAN (FOR YOUR FAMILY AND FRIENDS WHO ARE NOT KETOGENIC)

Maple Syrup

We aren't talking about your bottle of Mrs. Butterworth's. Instead, we are talking about 100 percent pure organic maple syrup. What makes this a much better alternative to traditional sugar is the fact that it contains good-for-you minerals like zinc and inflammation-fighting polyphenol antioxidants. And since it's sourced straight from tree sap, it goes through minimal processing to reach its conventional form. The darker the maple syrup, the better, because it contains higher amounts of antioxidants—up to twenty-four different kinds!

Honey

This is one of the best options when you need to add a little sweetness to your life. Honey's benefits are enormous, as long as you purchase it in its raw, unpasteurized, unfiltered form. It contains a wide range of powerful antioxidants like polyphenols, which have been shown to help combat cancer and promote heart health. It is also great for fighting off sickness since it still contains bee pollen, which has been shown to boost the immune system.

Manuka honey from New Zealand is the absolute best raw honey you can buy, because its nutritional content is so much higher than that of regular raw honey and it has intensive antimicrobial properties.

Molasses

This sweetener is made by boiling raw sugar down to remove the sucrose. This leaves behind the thick syrup we know as molasses. Blackstrap molasses is the most nutrient-dense form of molasses and is achieved by processing the syrup three times to remove as much sucrose as possible.

Dates

These sweet fruits are completely unprocessed and can be eaten fresh or dried or puréed into a paste to add to many different recipes. Since they are high in fructose, it is still important to keep their intake to a minimum.

Coconut Sugar and Nectar

These sweeteners are derived from the coconut blossoms of the coconut tree, not the coconut itself. Overall this is still a better option than regular sugar because it does contain a small amount of nutrients like zinc, potassium, and short-chain fatty acids. But you'd have to eat a lot to make a difference, so you'd be better off with completely natural options since this sweetener is still processed.

Coconut sugar contains inulin fiber, which has been shown to help improve diabetic health, because it helps to slow the absorption of glucose and keep blood-sugar levels balanced.

THE KETOTARIAN-APPROVED SWEETENERS

Last but surely not least, here are the options to turn to if you need to sweeten things up a bit.

Stevia

A zero-calorie low-glycemic sweetener that's also natural? It sounds almost too good to be true—and it kind of is. It all depends on what kind of stevia you are buying. Make sure you are getting raw organic stevia; otherwise, in conventional stevia brands, which may be heavily processed and are often bleached, you're still exposing yourself to other additives.

Sugar Alcohols

Often found in "sugar-free" foods, these would include sorbitol, mannitol, and xylitol and are derived through chemically processing the carbohydrates found in fruits and berries. These don't even have to be included on a product label unless it is specifically labeled "sugar-free." Unlike other sugar-free sweeteners that have zero calories, sugar alcohols do contain up to three calories per gram. Along with stevia, these sugar alcohols are still decent options for people looking for natural sugar-free options.

However, they don't work for everyone. Sugar alcohols have a laxative effect and can seriously flare up digestive problems like IBS and SIBO. Your body does not completely absorb these, and they end up fermenting in the large intestine, which can cause gas and bloating.

Monk Fruit

Like stevia and sugar alcohols, monk or luo han guo fruit is another low-carb sweetener option. It's fermented from the pulp of the fruit, which removes the sugars but leaves a residual sweet flavor. Used for hundreds of years in Asian countries where it is harvested, monk fruit contains beneficial antioxidants called mogrosides. Because of this, monk fruit has been used as a natural anti-inflammatory tool for centuries in Chinese medicine. You have to be aware of what kind you are purchasing, because some commercially available options have additives. So, read the labels and stick with pure monk fruit. And just like sugar alcohols such as xylitol, too much luo han guo can trigger stomach issues in some people.

5 | practical ketotarian:
Eating Out, Food Swaps, and Snack Ideas

how to eat out, ketotarian style

When going Ketotarian, many people are worried that they'll never be able to go to a restaurant again if they're going to lead this new healthy life. That just isn't true. You don't have to stay at home and live in a bubble to live a health-conscious life. I want to empower you with tips and tools to stay healthy when you are eating out.

- **Check out the menu online beforehand.** Most restaurants have their menu posted on their website. Perusing the online menu before you go will give you extra time to make an educated, healthy choice.

- **Keep the bread and chip baskets away.** That dreaded basket of grainy gratuitousness will be the antithesis of eating out healthily. Many people have a gluten or grain sensitivity and they don't even know it. Even if you don't have a detectable reactivity, the empty calories and refined carbohydrates of these nutrient-deficient foods will be an impediment to your fat-adapted life.

- **Bring your own sauces and dressings.** Many of my patients think I'm extreme with this tip, but I think it can be very helpful. Salad dressings and condiments like ketchup are typically filled with processed sugars; inflammatory oils like canola, soy, and corn; and artificial additives. Keeping healthy versions of these in your purse or bag will ensure that you're not unnecessarily exposing yourself to foods that have a simple, healthy alternative. Look for options that use olive or avocado oil, and avoid varieties with added sugars or bring your own!

- **Have a healthy snack before you go.** You may be thinking, "What's the point of eating out if I am going to eat before I go to the restaurant?" I'm not suggesting you eat a full meal beforehand, but a little healthy ketogenic snack will curb your craving to dive into the bread or chip basket when you first sit down.

- **Keep it simple.** When you're at a restaurant and are trying to eat healthily, typically the simpler the meal the better. A dish without added sauces or breading will avoid all the additives that are usually in them.

- **Speak up.** This is sometimes hard to do, but asking questions about the menu and mentioning that you are avoiding certain foods is essential to staying healthy when eating out. You are not hurting the server's feelings. This is your health we are talking about.

- **Ask for vegetables or a salad as a side substitute.** Instead of having fried foods or grains, ask for a side of steamed vegetables or a salad. And here's another easy tip you can use just about anywhere: ask for extra avocados or olives in your salad to pump up the healthy fats.

- **Ask what oil your food is cooked in.** Restaurants usually use cheaper oils, like canola or vegetable, to cook with. These oils, as you know already, are pro-inflammatory polyunsaturated omega-6 fats that have a low smoke point and are easily oxidized. I can't wait for the day when all restaurants use avocado or coconut oil, but for now, asking for a fat that can withstand heat will be your best option. Olive is a great option for cold uses like dressings, but extra virgin olive oil will oxidize easily when heated.

- **Support health-conscious restaurants.** A growing number of restaurants offer healthy, real-food options. Menus filled with delicious, healthy meals will make it so much more enjoyable for you! Seek them out in your area and tell them you stand with them by supporting their health-conscious business.

- **Do your best, then don't stress.** Use all of these tips, then let the rest go and enjoy yourself. You can't control everything, so give yourself grace. Your body is resilient and has survived this long, so don't stress. Be encouraged and go enjoy some good food.

ketotarian on the go

Whether you're on vacation, on the road, having a busy day, or just looking for something quick and convenient, look no further. Here are some ideas for easy snacks to have on hand.

- Shredded coconut with your favorite nuts
- MCT or coconut oil in tea, coffee, water, or smoothies
- Marine collagen in tea, coffee, water, or smoothies
- Coconut cream with berries

- Hard-boiled eggs
- Grain-free granola
- Avocado halves (you can salt, pepper, and drizzle with oil)
- Pickles
- Chia seed pudding
- Flax crackers

- Almond flour crackers
- Pumpkin seeds
- Olives
- Seaweed snacks
- Tigernuts
- Fat bombs
- Almond butter on celery

- Single-serving packets of almond butter, coconut oil, or avocado oil
- Salmon jerky
- Canned salmon
- Canned tuna
- Canned sardines
- Canned oysters

ketotarian food swaps

Considering the fact that about 90 cents of every dollar spent at the grocery store goes toward processed junk food, our culture needs a healthy intervention! And while the thought of cleaning up the fridge and pantry can be daunting, with many people putting off eating clean for another day, if you were waiting for the right time to start making healthier choices—it's now.

You are alive because of brilliant biochemistry, and the foods you eat instruct every facet of your health, feeding either health or disease. My job as a functional-medicine expert is not only to get to the root cause of health problems; it's to develop realistic and sustainable solutions to heal them. And when it comes to healthy eating, here's a secret: you don't have to eat like a rabbit or restrict yourself to only kale salads (no offense, kale lovers).

Instead, allow me to introduce you to the art of food hacking. Here are my favorite fun and easy alternatives to the world's most beloved meals. Let's transform your go-to comfort foods into nutrient-dense superfoods and start healing with meals— not medicine.

- Spaghetti squash, zucchini, or shirataki noodles instead of regular pasta
- Cauliflower rice instead of rice
- Nut cheese instead of dairy cheese
- Cauliflower hummus instead of hummus
- Mashed avocado instead of mayonnaise

- Chia seed pudding instead of oatmeal or cereal
- Grain-free flax and nut granola instead of cereal
- Coconut milk yogurt instead of dairy yogurt
- Coconut flakes instead of bread crumbs
- Mashed cauliflower instead of mashed potatoes

- Lettuce wraps instead of sandwiches
- Almond flour waffles or pancakes instead of conventional varieties
- Flax tortillas instead of corn or wheat tortillas
- Almond, chia, or flaxseed flour crackers instead of conventional crackers

- Flavored carbonated water instead of soda
- Carob, cacao, baker's chocolate, or dark chocolate instead of milk chocolate
- Coconut aminos instead of soy sauce
- Coconut whip instead of whipped cream

ketotarian superfoods of the land and sea

Now that we have covered the Ketotarian essentials, let's take it to the next level. I handpicked my favorite oceanic and terrestrial superfoods. These are all optional, so don't stress about trying all or any of them. Once you get the basics down, these are here to amplify your Ketotarian journey.

THE SEA

Wild-caught fish isn't the only food medicine of the sea that you can use in your Ketotarian plan. Here are eight other ways to harness some oceanic magic:

Spirulina and Blue-Green Algae

Spirulina and other blue-green algae are naturally found in freshwater and saltwater lakes around the world. Traditionally, blue-green algae were used by ancient civilizations in Mexico and Africa as a superfood. And now you can find them in powder form at your local health food store!

What they do for you

Spirulina is jam-packed with tons of benefits; it contains three times the protein of beef and all nine essential amino acids (the ones your body can't make that you need to get from food). Spirulina also has more calcium than milk, and its chlorophyll content makes it super detoxifying. These blue-green algae are also a great source of those uber-important bioavailable omega fats if you decide not to eat fish or eggs.

How to use them

It's blue-green algae that gives the mermaid and unicorn lattes their brilliant aquatic hues. Even Starbucks' sugar-laden, short-lived unicorn frap took advantage of spirulina to get its beautiful color. Try mixing a teaspoon or two of blue majik algae into your own healthy elixirs, teas, and smoothies! Check out some of my favorite recipes in Chapter 8.

Sea Vegetables

With exotic names like hijiki, nori, dulse, kombu, kelp, arame, Irish moss, and alaria esculenta, seaweeds have been consumed in Asia, New Zealand, Ireland, and other island cultures for thousands of years. Technically also types of algae, sea vegetables all have a unique taste, look, and texture.

What they do for you

Sea vegetables are one of the most diverse mineral sources on earth. These green superfoods are full of B vitamins, vitamin C, vitamin K, magnesium, and eighteen amino acids. These vegetables of the ocean are also good plant sources for omega fats. Sea vegetables are also considered the most effective way to get the ultra important mineral iodine, which is needed to make your thyroid hormones. Sea vegetables also contain compounds called fucans that have various anti-inflammatory properties and have been shown to improve blood sugar numbers in people with type 2 diabetes.

How to use them
You can soak sea vegetables in soups, sprinkle flakes in your salads, use the sheets as wraps, or blend them in smoothies.

Pearl

Yes, that kind of pearl. This valued product from oysters has been used in traditional Asian medicine for generations. Crushed to a fine powder, pearl is used in skin care products and supplements, touted as a secret to ageless beauty.

What it does for you
Pearl is the oceanic adaptogen and is often used for its calming and mood-regulating effects. Calcium-rich pearl also contains magnesium, amino acids, and a variety of minerals, making it a super beauty food for radiant skin.

How to use it
Pearl has a mild taste, so it goes great in just about everything. I use a teaspoon in smoothies and elixirs, but you can even put it in some healthy baked goods!

Marine Phytoplankton

This specific kind of microalga is considered the most important plant in the world. This is because it provides the earth with over 90 percent of its oxygen—more than all the forests in the world combined! But marine phytoplankton is not only an important source of oxygen; it's a critical food source for ocean life and humans, too.

What it does for you
Few foods on this earth provide the raw materials for our bodies to make new cells and sustain the ones we have, but marine phytoplankton is one of them. It contains

all nine amino acids that the body cannot make on its own, along with the essential omega fats, vitamins A and C and a variety of B vitamins, and trace minerals. Think of it as pure food for your cells.

How to use it

Unless you're going to wade around the ocean lopping up microalgae, the best way to get phytoplankton is through supplementation.

Sea Salt

Salt from our most pristine oceans is actually an amazing superfood—nothing like conventional table salt. Hawaiian sea salt is a beautiful red color from volcanic rock, Italian sea salt is harvested off the Mediterranean coast of Sicily, Celtic salt off the coast of France, and beautiful pink Himalayan sea salt is harvested from ancient seabeds, originally formed from marine fossil deposits over 250 million years ago.

What it does for you

These salts have a wide array of minerals that aid in optimal immune, hormone, and electrolyte balance.

How to use it

Use these superfood salts like you would your run-of-the-mill salts. Sprinkle them on just about anything when you want to add more flavor. Another way to use the power of sea salts is to simulate the ocean by drawing yourself a detox bath. Just pour two cups of one of these salts into your bath and soak up the healing properties straight through your skin.

Krill Oil

Krill are tiny crustaceans found in every ocean, and there are more of these little guys on the planet than any other creature. To put this into perspective, if you were to weigh the population of any animal on earth, even humans, krill would still weigh the most.

What it does for you

Most of us are lacking healthy fats, specifically the omega-3s, which contributes to health problems like depression, heart disease, arthritis, and inflammation. Krill oil has been found, in many ways, to be superior to conventional fish oil as it contains fifty times as much of the powerful antioxidant astaxanthin. The beneficial phospholipids phosphatidylcholine and phosphatidylserine—needed for optimal cellular, hormone, brain, and nerve health—are also present in this unique oil.

How to use it

Krill oil is usually sold in capsules, and you would take them like any supplement. I'm a big fan of Neptune krill oil (NKO) and take it daily for two reasons. First, it's one of the most nutrient-dense kinds of krill oil, and second, I think anything with the word *Neptune* in front of it sounds cool.

Marine Collagen

Putting grass-fed collagen powder in lattes and coffee is definitely a health trend, but one lesser-known collagen option is marine collagen from wild-caught fish.

What it does for you

One of the cleanest, most bioavailable sources of protein, marine collagen is also a great way to promote healthy skin, hair, and joints. Rich in glycine, collagen is also great for supporting optimal gut and immune health.

How to use it

You will most commonly find marine collagen in powdered form. Try adding a scoop to your favorite almond or coconut milk latte.

Magnesium Salt

The ancient Zechstein Sea—a geological formation in northern Europe—is rich with magnesium salt. This type of magnesium has been protected, deep within the Zechstein Seabed at a depth of 2,000 meters beneath the earth's crust, from the toxins of our modern world.

What it does for you

Magnesium is responsible for hundreds of different crucial pathways in your body. Your hormones, brain, and heart depend on optimal magnesium levels, and most of us are deficient!

How to use it

My favorite way to get this type of magnesium is from magnesium oil spray. This is one of the most bioavailable ways to ensure optimal magnesium levels.

THE LAND

Bee Pollen

Bee pollen is a beautiful food from flowers and bees. When bees collect nectar for honey, they cover their legs with pollen. Bee pollen is collected when they return to their hive when a screen gently scrapes the pollen off their legs. Native Americans were known to wear pouches containing pollen around their necks for long journeys. The father of medicine, Hippocrates, prescribed bee pollen as a revered food medicine.

What it does for you

Bee pollen is rich in antioxidants, minerals, vitamins (especially high levels of B vitamins), and essential amino acids (approximately 40 percent protein).

How to use it

You can sprinkle this yummy food on coconut yogurt, blend it in smoothies, or eat it off a spoon.

Adaptogens

The adaptogenic kingdom is composed of plant and earth medicines that balance out your hormones and help calm stress levels—but there's so much more. Your body's stress system, the sympathetic nervous system, controls hundreds of pathways that are responsible for inflammation. And this is important because the hectic, crazy, modern world we live in can leave us feeling exhausted, inflamed, irritable, hangry, and emotionally spent—all of which can lead to hormonal problems like adrenal fatigue, low sex drive, and thyroid problems.

Adaptogens give the stress system (and you) a big proverbial cuddle—keeping inflammation levels in check. And because chronic inflammation is linked to many of the common health problems we see today, the medical literature has found adaptogens to have other far-reaching health benefits, including the following:

- Lowering cortisol levels
- Regenerating brain cells
- Alleviating depression and anxiety
- Protecting heart health
- Protecting the liver
- Preventing and fighting cancer
- Lowering cholesterol
- Protecting against radiation
- Balancing the immune system
- Decreasing fatigue

Take-home message: Adaptogens are badass. All of these little guys fight inflammation and generally have a knack for bringing some zen to your adrenal, thyroid, and sex hormones. But each adaptogen also has its own special set of skills. Here are some of my favorite adaptogens and what you should know about each:

Ginseng: the pick-me-up
Asian White, Asian Red, American White: the ginseng varieties are great for people who want an extra boost of energy without the jitters of caffeine. I love using ginseng for jet lag.

Rhodiola: the stress calmer
Rhodiola rosea can be a great tool to use for people struggling with adrenal fatigue and fibromyalgia. But take note: if you are extra sensitive, Rhodiola can keep you up at night.

Schisandra: the adrenal balancer

Another super adrenal supporter, this berry is one I used on a regular basis during my journey recovering from adrenal fatigue.

Shilajit: the sex hormone igniter

People with low libido or sex hormone imbalance can often benefit from shilajit. The name of this Ayurvedic herb translates as "conqueror of mountains and destroyer of weakness." Sounds good to me.

Ashwagandha: the thyroid and mood master

A superstar adaptogen, this popular herb is a great tool in supporting optimal thyroid function and mitigating mood swings. Ashwagandha is also a nightshade, which some people with autoimmune conditions can't handle.

Maca: the energizer

Maca is a great way to boost energy and also calm anxiety naturally. Maca is a rich source of vitamin C, making it great for boosting the immune system. There are three types of maca powders: red, yellow, and black. Red maca is the sweetest and mildest tasting. Yellow maca is the least sweet, and black maca is somewhere in between the two.

Holy Basil (Tulsi): the memory booster

I find holy basil to be great for people with brain fog, gently working to increase cognitive function. It is also great for bloating and gas.

Ho Shou Wu: the libido pumper-upper

Another great tool for people with a low sex drive, this herb has been used for thousands of years in Chinese medicine.

Mucuna pruriens: nature's chill pill

This adaptogenic bean extract is jam-packed with L-DOPA, the precursor to the neurotransmitter dopamine. I take this daily as it helps with my focus and calms me down during my busy day.

Eleuthero: the battery pack

If you are dragging through the day, this is another way to optimize your energy levels. Extra stressful week? Eleuthero is your guy.

Adaptogenic mushrooms

Within the adaptogenic kingdom there is also an extra-special group of medicinal mushrooms that offer some of the same hormone-balancing benefits as the preceding adaptogens and some extra immune-boosting qualities too:

- Chaga
- Himematsutake
- Turkey Tail
- Reishi
- Shiitake
- Lion's Mane
- Cordyceps

How to use adaptogens

Adaptogens are typically sold in powdered form, and because they each offer their own unique benefit, I am a fan of using blends in elixirs and smoothies. Have fun as you experiment to find the right mix for your needs.

supplements to consider for your ketotarian lifestyle

Food is foundational for the Ketotarian. You can't supplement your way out of a poor diet. With that said, many people can take their health to the next level with targeted use of supplements.

There are so many supplements on the market that it can be overwhelming to know what the uses and benefits are and which ones are right for you. As a functional-medicine practitioner, I typically see a wide range of well-intentioned but unnecessary options. This can lead to an ever-expanding supplement graveyard. Often there are really only a handful of vitamins and supplements that need to be considered to optimize your overall health. So, let's cut through the confusion. Here is your essential guide to vitamins, their uses and benefits, and how to incorporate them into your Ketotarian routine.

VITAMIN D

No other vitamin can hold a candle to vitamin D and its importance. Since vitamin D is fat-soluble, it acts more like a hormone than a vitamin by regulating hundreds of uber-important pathways in your body. Besides your thyroid hormones, this vitamin is the only other thing every single cell of your body needs in order to function properly. Vitamin D is also known as the sunshine vitamin; your body makes vitamin D by absorbing sunlight and then converting it to a usable form. We can't get the amount we truly need from food alone, so supplementing is key so that we don't become deficient, especially if you live far from the equator or in a place where sunny days aren't always the norm.

Dosage

In functional medicine we aim for an optimal range between 60 and 80 ng/mL. Depending on where your starting levels are, anywhere between 2,000 and 6,000 IU is an adequate amount per day. Make sure to test your vitamin D levels to find out your starting point, and retest to gauge how your vitamin D level optimization is going.

How to Incorporate

Since vitamin D is fat-soluble, take advantage of vitamin synergy by combining it with other fat-soluble vitamins, such as A and K2. This will help make it more bioavailable and balanced. It's also a great idea to take them with fatty foods like avocado, olive oil, wild-caught fish, and coconut to increase their bioavailability.

MAGNESIUM

This mineral is needed for over three hundred crucial biochemical reactions in your body, including the regulation of neurotransmitter functions. Up to 80 percent of the population is deficient in this nutrient, leading to problems with sleep, anxiety, migraines, and brain fog. Most deficiencies come from a poor diet or gut problems, making magnesium absorption difficult.

There are many different forms of magnesium, so let's break down the best.

Magnesium citrate is the most commonly found in supplement form and is a good option. Magnesium glycinate is more easily absorbed by the body, and magnesium threonate seems promising for more neurological support. Magnesium oil is another great way to boost this vital nutrient.

Dosage
350 mg per day.

How to Incorporate
Taking magnesium right before bed is often best as it promotes better sleep by relaxing muscles and helping the calming neurotransmitter, GABA, in your brain.

PROBIOTICS

As Hippocrates said, "All disease begins in the gut." Science is finally catching up, with research showing that the gut is the foundation for almost all aspects of your health—regardless of whether you are having digestive symptoms. Your gut microbiome contains trillions of bacteria, and an imbalance of good bacteria can affect everything from your weight to your hormones. While it is important to include probiotic-rich foods such as kefir, kimchi, sauerkraut, and kombucha into your diet, depending on your level of gut permeability, you may need an additional boost from a probiotic supplement.

Dosage
At least 10 billion CFU per day.

How to Incorporate
To really amp up the effects of your probiotics, include enough prebiotic foods, such as garlic, asparagus, and onions, into your diet. These fibrous foods act as fuel for your probiotics by helping facilitate the growth of good gut bacteria. When choosing a probiotic, make sure to take one that includes strains of *Lactobacilli* and *Bifidobacteria*. These two strains are shown to reduce inflammation. I am also a fan of soil-based probiotics (SBOs) to further support rich bacterial diversity.

OMEGA-3 FISH OIL

Healthy fat is essential for optimal brain health, as your brain itself is composed of about 60 percent fat, so depriving your body of fat can contribute to brain fog, fatigue, depression, and anxiety. So if you're not getting enough healthy fats, specifically enough from wild-caught seafood, you might want to consider an omega-3 fish oil supplement. Omega fats can be found in plant sources such as flax, but it's not easily used by our bodies because it must be converted into DHA or EPA, which is an inefficient process. Because of this, I suggest getting your omega fats from fish oil from salmon, cod liver, or sardines.

Dosage

2,250 mg EPA/750 mg DHA per day.

How to Incorporate

If you're eating more omega-6 fatty acids (like those found in certain oils like safflower oil)—which can increase inflammation throughout the body—try taking fish oil to reduce the inflammatory effects.

TURMERIC

Inflammation is at the center of every chronic health problem today. Turmeric is a powerful anti-inflammatory tool to have in your health arsenal. Whether you are taking turmeric or curcumin (the powerful antioxidant found within turmeric), you can begin to win the battle against inflammation.

Dosage

For those looking for inflammation maintenance, 2 grams per day is a good start, but as much as 10 grams per day may be needed to drive down higher levels of inflammation.

How to Incorporate

Unless you know that you are currently struggling with chronic high levels of inflammation, this is not necessarily something you need to be including in your routine every single day. For the average person eating a healthy diet, cooking with this spice is more than enough to reap the benefits. Piperine, the compound found in black pepper, increases the bioavailability of curcumin by 2,000 percent, so find a supplement that includes this compound.

VITAMIN C

This vitamin is most commonly associated with the common cold, as it's a powerful immune booster found to reduce symptoms by up to 30 percent.

Dosage

1,000 to 4,000 mg per day to boost your immune system and promote healthy skin.

How to Incorporate

Combining vitamin C with zinc can increase its immune-boosting properties. You can easily find powdered supplements that you can mix with water to take with you for when you start to feel a little less than 100 percent.

ZINC

Your body has no way to store this important mineral, so it is important to make sure you're getting it through your diet or supplementation. Its main role is to help your body increase white blood cells and fight off infection, and it also assists with the release of antibodies. Deficiency has been linked to increased instances of sickness, so it is no wonder you often find zinc as a common ingredient in the cold and flu aisle of your pharmacy.

Dosage

15 to 30 mg per day. Pregnant women should aim for 12 mg per day since it's essential for normal fetal development.

How to Incorporate

If you're eating a healthy, well-rounded diet, you should be getting in the proper amount of zinc per day without needing a supplement. But if getting over a cold quickly is your goal, supplementing at least 75 mg per day has been shown to greatly reduce cold duration and symptoms so you can get back to optimal health.

METHYLATED B COMPLEX

B vitamins are the fuel behind methylation, the ongoing biochemical process that helps keep you alive and healthy by assisting in your body's ability to properly detox. There are many types of B vitamins, so it's important to get in a well-rounded amount of each.

Dosage

400 to 800 mcg methylfolate (B_9) and 1,000 mcg methylcobalamin (B_{12}) per day.

How to Incorporate

The best B vitamin supplement would be a B-complex vitamin containing methylated B vitamins, especially if you have methylation impairments like the MTHFR gene mutation. Look for activated B vitamins like B9 L-methylfolate (L-5-MTHF), B_6 pyridoxyl-5-phosphate (P5P), and B_{12} versions (such as adenosyl B_{12}, cyano B_{12}, hydroxycobalamin B_{12}, or methyl B_{12}).

VITAMIN A

Vitamin A is essential for equipping you with a strong immune system. And vitamin A deficiency has also been linked to autoimmune diseases, which are on the rise in a major way.

Look for vitamin A sources from either whole-food sources like fish liver oil or retinyl palmitate.

Dosage

2,000 to 10,000 IU per day.

VITAMIN K2

Vitamin K2 is effective at inhibiting the pro-inflammatory iNOS pathway. Unfortunately, K2 is one of the most common nutrient deficiencies in the Western diet. There are several types of K2, but I suggest looking for the MK-4 version. MK-4 regulates gene expression in specific ways that no other form of vitamin K does. MK-4 plays an exclusive role in cancer protection and sexual health.

Dosage

100 to 200 mcg per day.

How to Incorporate

Taking these fat-soluble vitamins together with vitamin D will help keep your levels from going too high as well as making vitamin D more bioavailable to your body. Because these are fat-soluble, they are absorbed best by taking them with a fat-containing meal such as avocado, salmon, or just a bit of butter or coconut oil added to whatever you're cooking.

Remember, food is your best medicine. You can't supplement your way out of a poor diet. Supplements are just that— supplementary.

In summary, you can take many of these nutrients in a multivitamin, and some you will need to take separately to get the dosage I'm recommending. Remember, food is your best medicine. You can't supplement your way out of a poor diet. Supplements are just that—supplementary.

Of course, not everyone needs to or should incorporate each of these vitamins and supplements into their wellness routine. It's always important to take your individual needs and health case into consideration. Working with a functional-medicine practitioner can help you determine what exactly you are lacking, and therefore what you should be supplementing with.

ketotarian-approved protein powders

Many of my patients love protein powders. You can add them to your morning smoothie for a quick, satisfying breakfast or even add them to baked goods to bulk up the nutritional value.

For all of these options, read the label. It's not always the protein itself that's a problem—often it is the added ingredients that are the issue. Watch out for sugars and fillers, and always go for organic with the fewest added ingredients possible.

And remember, whole, real food should be your primary source of protein, but protein powders can be a nice option if you are on the go, want to mix things up, working out, or making your favorite smoothie recipe. Don't forget to add healthy fats like avocado, coconut oil, coconut milk, ghee, or organic, pasture-raised egg yolks to your smoothies. Make your real-food smoothie a vehicle for green veggies and health fats.

SACHA INCHI

Also known as the Inca peanut, this seed found in Peru is a complete plant protein containing every single essential amino acid at 9 grams of protein per serving. Its high omega fat content makes it a perfect source for helping healthy hormones. Since it is plant-based, though, it will not be as bioavailable as collagen. But for those wanting a plant-based complete protein without grains, this is probably my favorite choice.

HEMP

Compared to other plant- or animal-based protein powders, this is one of the lowest in protein content. While hemp is filled with other great factors such as fiber and omega fat, which is needed for a happy and healthy gut and brain, it contains only about 30 to 50 percent protein by weight compared to 90 to 100 percent of other choices. And not only is the protein content lackluster, but the amount it does have is less bioavailable than animal or pea proteins. This type of protein has few negative hormonal side effects. In fact, since it provides loads of vitamin E, fiber, iron, and essential fatty acids, it can be a great choice since your body can't produce these kinds of fats on its own, so they must be part of your regular diet.

PEA

Derived from yellow split peas, this protein powder contains all nine essential amino acids. However, three of them are in very small amounts, so it may still be necessary to pair it with a complementary protein. Studies show that it can help keep you full for longer, which can make it perfect for adding to morning smoothies. Some people don't tolerate legumes, even podlike legumes like peas, so for these people, pea protein can throw off their digestion and hormones. If your stomach is at all irritated when you consume legumes, avoid pea protein.

PUMPKIN SEED

Pumpkin lovers can take their obsession to a whole new level with the addition of pumpkin seed protein powder. It's considered a complete plant protein with all nine amino acids at 12 grams of protein per 1-cup serving. Because pumpkin seed protein is high in healthy fats (with 12 grams per cup), it is good for keeping hormones balanced, maintaining a healthy brain, and providing long-lasting sustainable energy. Some people don't tolerate seeds, so for these people, this is a no-go.

SOY

We can't talk about protein sources without mentioning the ever-controversial soy. Soy protein comes from dehulled and defatted soybeans, which are then further processed to achieve three different forms: soy concentrates, soy isolates, and soy flour. For anyone who is estrogen dominant (mostly women, but also some men), soy can potentially be a problem. If you are going to go for soy, make sure you are looking for non-GMO varieties.

COLLAGEN

Found in our skin, cartilage, tendons, bones, ligaments, blood vessels, and more, this protein is needed for a healthy metabolism as well as our own collagen production. It is composed of three amino acids: proline, glycine, and hydroxyproline. Your body produces all three but not enough to be beneficial, so supplementation through diet is important. Our bodies need about 15 grams of glycine a day—but the average person typically consumes only about 3 grams. You can get collagen in two different forms that are Ketotarian compliant, both containing different subtypes of collagen:

Fish Collagen

Also referred to as marine collagen, this is another one of my all-time favorites. Not only does it provide the essential Type I collagen, but it is also one of the most bio-available because the collagen peptides are smaller particles.

Eggshell Membrane Collagen

This kind of collagen contains both Type I and Type V collagen, which work together for healthy joint and connective tissues and help encourage muscle growth.

EGG WHITE

This is a highly bioavailable protein option that is used as the standard for determining the bioavailability of other sources. It's also fantastic because it provides all of the necessary amino acids your body needs. The albumin in egg whites can be a source of inflammation for some, but if you can tolerate eggs, this is one of the better options.

6

first steps:
How to Get Started on Your Ketotarian Journey

Now that you know what to eat and what to avoid, let's jump into how to get started on your Ketotarian lifestyle. In order to maximize your success in Ketotarian living, you need to be intentional and prepared to make these healthy changes. Consulting thousands of patients over the years, I know what works and what doesn't, and I have heard just about every question there is. Yes, this change may seem overwhelming at first, but I'll cut through the confusion and keep it simple.

Remember back to when you learned how to ride a bike or drive a car, yet now these things are second nature. So too will your plant-based ketogenic eating be once you get the hang of it. Before you know it, you'll be throwing off those training wheels. So, let's get started!

For each step, I will tell you exactly what to do, and I will also give you some "keep it simple" options throughout if you want to take things slowly.

step 1. food logging and becoming mindful of the foods you are eating

The ultimate goal for your new Ketotarian lifestyle is to make sure you are eating quality and healing keto plant-based foods. However, it is so important to find the right ratios of macronutrients that will help you become fat-adapted and enhance how you feel. There are plenty of keto food-tracking apps that you can download easily on your phone. Keto diet logging apps make it simple, tracking how much fat, protein, and carbs you have eaten and how much you need for the day. So, put that calculator and pencil away and use technology to your advantage. And remember, once you get the hang of it, this will be second nature. You will know what your body loves, hates, and needs in order to thrive.

Food logging is not meant to make you become obsessive about food but to help you grow in awareness of what you are eating. Some people find that food tracking long term is helpful, while others don't need to once they get the hang of what their body loves and where they feel the best.

Once you become aware of the macronutrients in your food (where your fuel is coming from), the goal is to just eat until satiety—in other words, until you're satisfied, not until you're full.

KEEP-IT-SIMPLE OPTION

If the healthy foods on the Ketotarian food list are new to you, give yourself grace and patience. One option for you is to ease into it. Spend the first two weeks just eating from the allowed food list. Don't worry too much about the serving sizes or tracking your macronutrients, just eat from the foods on the allowed list until you're satisfied. Don't log your food intake for these two weeks if you don't want to; just keep it simple. Spend these first two weeks getting used to these healthy food choices, clearing out your pantry and fridge of anything that isn't on the allowed list. After your two-week healthy transition, just start at step 1. You've got this.

If the allowed food list doesn't seem like a foreign language, you can jump right into Step 1.

step 2. personalizing your macronutrients

CARBS

To make this as easy as possible, your carbohydrate intake will be less than 55 grams net carbs (total carbs minus the fiber) from real plant food carbs every day. As you are starting out, I suggest starting at under 25 grams net carbs a day and working your way up from there over the first month. By starting on the lower end of the carbohydrate range, you can become keto-adapted more quickly. Once you are in nutritional ketosis, you can slowly increase your daily intake to a max of 55 grams net carbs a day to find how many carbohydrates you can eat while staying in nutritional ketosis. This is your personal Ketotarian plan, which means that adjustments can be made to fit your needs and where you feel your best. Healthy carbs will make up 5 to 15 percent of your caloric intake.

Keep-it-simple option

Most keto food-logging apps can track net carbs as well as total carbs, which takes all the guesswork out. Another way to keep total vs net carbs simple is to not count non-starchy green vegetable carbs and avocado at all (because they are so low in carbs and so high in fiber) and only count fruit and starchy vegetables like sweet potatoes in your total carb count.

PROTEIN

Protein is made of amino acids, which are necessary for a lot of pathways to keep us healthy and strong. They do a lot of work by carrying nutrients to the cells and play a big role in regulation of the body's tissues and organs.[1] We need protein to fuel the muscles in our body, but exactly how much do we need? Remember that a healthy ketogenic diet is high in fat, low in carbohydrates, and *moderate* in protein.

One common pitfall that I find among those eating the average ketogenic or low-carb diet is overdoing it on the protein. Excess protein intake during a ketogenic diet could possibly keep us from getting into ketosis by stimulating gluconeogenesis, a process in which glucose is created in the body when you eat more protein than you actually need.

Eating too much protein has been linked to an increase of mTOR, the pathway that is responsible for an acceleration of cell division, which leads to accelerated aging and activation of cancer. Eating too little protein is bad for our health as well, leading to growth failure, loss of muscle mass, decreased immunity, weakening of the heart and respiratory system, and more. Protein intake is imperative when it comes to a healthy keto lifestyle. You want to be in your protein sweet spot. For most of us, I suggest between 0.5 and 1 gram of protein per pound of lean body mass (not your total body weight). Your lean body weight or mass (LBM) is the amount of weight on your body that isn't fat. There are many calculators online that easily allow you to calculate your LBM. High-endurance athletes, some seniors, and pregnant or breast-feeding moms may need to go to 0.9 to 1.5 grams of protein per pound of lean body mass. Overall, your daily protein intake will be 15 to 30 percent of your overall calorie intake.

Remember, keto diet food-tracking apps will help with this if math isn't your thing.

FATS

Okay, so now it's time to talk about how much fat you really need. If we look at the percentages of our carbohydrates and protein, then the rest of the foods you are going to eat are, you guessed it, healthy fats. Your caloric intake will consist of anywhere from 60 to 75 percent (maybe a little more) of fat per day.

step 3. checking in on your ketosis

In order to reset your metabolism to be fat-adapted, we first have to get your body into nutritional ketosis. You may be thinking, "What is the difference between the two?" When you first start eating Ketotarian, your body will begin producing ketones and draining glycogen (stored sugar) stores, but it isn't relying on fat as its primary energy source. On the other hand, when you are fat-adapted, your body will produce those ketones and use fat as its main source for fuel even when you eat carbohydrates. This is the metabolic flexibility that will allow you to eventually play around with your macronutrients and find your unique threshold of carbohydrate and protein tolerance to see where the body finally switches from sugar-burning to fat-burning mode. If you are eating too many carbohydrates, your body will always choose to burn those first for energy. Remember, like kindling on a fire, sugar is the quickest and easiest to burn. However, when you are fat-adapted it's like the sugar-burning switch is flipped off and only switches back on once we've stepped over our own individual threshold. We have to test our ketones so that we know our bodies are burning them. There are a few different ways to test for this because they are different types of ketones in the body: acetate, acetoacetate, and beta-hydroxybutryate.

- Blood Meter

- Breath Meter

- Urine Testing

BLOOD METER

A blood ketone meter is one of the most common and most accurate tools when testing for ketosis. Similar to a blood glucose meter, the ketone meter uses ketone testing strips to identify the levels of ketones in the blood. The key ketone used by the body, beta-hydroxybutryate (BHB), is carried through the blood so it can get to the cells to be used for energy and fuel. Because blood ketone levels in our body are not easily affected by different variables (like ketones in the breath or urine are), this makes blood ketone testing the most accurate representation of how many ketones we are producing. If you are already used to testing your blood sugar, this test is basically the same process. You may even have a meter that can test sugars and ketones. What's great about this test is that it gives you a measurable source of ketones in the blood. There is no guesswork in it or having to correlate a shade of color with the level of ketones, as in urine testing. Straightforward and to the point. When you are in nutritional ketosis your levels should consistently be between 0.5 and 1.0 mmol. As you become more fat-adapted, those numbers will rise to 1.5 to 3.0 mmol. Remember that there is no magical number within that range where you need to be. Your optimal level is the level where you feel best and can reach your goals.

Nutritional ketosis is 0.5 to 1.0 mmol

Optimal ketosis is 1.5 to 3.0 mmol

Higher ketones don't necessarily mean better. Are you in the zone or not? That's what is important.

The downside to this test is that even though it is considered the most accurate, it is not the most cost-effective as the strips are a few dollars each. If you are testing every day, it can add up.

BREATH METER

A breath analyzer is another great tool used to test ketones. Because of its small size, breath acetone (BrAce) diffuses into the lungs and we can measure it in our breath.[2]

When you breathe out, BrAce increases.[3] Multiple studies have shown that acetone in the breath strongly correlates to the BHB in the blood. The acetone is recognized through a breath meter that will measure and use color or numbers to tell you the level of ketones your body is making. This noninvasive technique can be more appealing to those who do not want to have to prick their finger every day, it is a reliable test, and the breath meter is a reusable tool that you pay for once, no strips needed. One potential drawback is that breath ketones can easily be affected by things like alcohol consumption and water intake. These are all things to consider when deciding which tool will best fit into your goals and vision for success.

URINE TESTING

The third tool for measuring ketones is urine test strips. These are pretty simple and straightforward. Urine test strips measure excess acetoacetate ketones that have been excreted through the urine. These tests are super easy; you just pee on the strip and after 30 to 45 seconds it will turn a shade of color so you can see the level of ketones in the urine. The shade is not an exact measurement of ketones like the blood ketone meter results. Studies have suggested that urine testing for ketones is best done early in the morning or hours after dinner late in the evening.[4]

The urine test strips are convenient because they are a cheap, easy, and noninvasive tool for looking at ketones in the urine during the transition into becoming keto-adapted, but long term I wouldn't use urine strips to gauge your nutritional ketosis.

The problem with urine testing is that as we become more fat-adapted, our body will be able to more efficiently use these ketones, which means we will not be excreting as much. Also, urinating ketones doesn't mean you're burning them in the first place. We just know your body is great at peeing them out! Other factors can cause urine testing to vary, such as electrolyte levels and hydration. Because of all this, urine strips are not a very accurate way to gauge your metabolic state.

Other Ways to Tell You Are in Ketosis

- Your fasting blood sugar levels are below 80 mL/dL and you still feel energized.

- You have none of that "hangry" business.

- You have increased mental clarity and focus.

- You have more sustained energy throughout the day.

- You do not want or need to snack.

- You can go a few hours without wanting to eat or can skip meals easily.

TO TEST OR NOT TO TEST?

Although testing for ketones while you're living Ketotarian is a good idea, especially at the beginning, you also want to listen to what your body is telling you. Plenty of natural changes happen as you become fat-adapted. Everyone is different, but a few signs of this metabolic shift are common. Our bodies burn fat more slowly than carbs, so you should feel more steadily energized throughout the day, with an increase in mental clarity. Because you aren't relying on carbohydrates as your primary fuel source anymore, you should have a better regulation of our blood sugar. You can even have lower blood sugars, but you feel like you're on top of the world and don't feel weak and shaky. You may find yourself able to skip meals and fast easily. And you can say good-bye to that hangry feeling because the satiety you will be feeling from the increase in healthy fats will take care of that as well. Pay attention to what your body is telling you.

WHAT TO DO IF YOU'RE NOT GETTING INTO KETOSIS

Can't get into ketosis? If you are testing your ketones from blood, breath, or urine and you are not in ketosis, here is your checklist to make sure you are doing everything you need to do.

1. Tweak your macronutrients and stay hydrated.

As you are starting out on your plant-based ketogenic lifestyle, I definitely suggest that you track your food intake until you get the hang of it and you have a routine. Remember, this is not "dieting" or becoming obsessive about food. It's just a way to become conscious of the foods you are eating and how they fuel your body. Also, there is no need to get a calculator. There are many keto or general food-tracking phone apps and developments in the wellness-tech industry that will do all of the calculations for you. Once this is second nature and you have your go-to foods, you don't necessarily have to log if you are hitting your goals and you feel great. Also, make sure you are drinking at least eight glasses of water every day. Proper hydration helps your overall metabolism function optimally.

Remember:

• Keep carbs low (25 to 55 grams net carbs as you get started from real plant foods)

• Moderate your protein

• Increase your healthy fats

2. Try lowering your carbs for a while.

Some people are extra sensitive to carbs. People with insulin resistance and other inflammatory issues may have to do under 25 grams net carbs to get into ketosis. Once you are in ketosis you can slowly increase your carbs, testing to see where your individual carb tolerance is.

3. Eat until satiety.

Ketotarian is focused on satiating, nutrient-dense foods. It's important to eat enough foods until you are satisfied. Remember, don't fear food; it's your friend and fuel. Conversely, be sure not to eat beyond satisfaction, either. If you are used to overeating, it can take time to become conscious and connected with your body and how foods make it feel. Chew slowly and be present while you eat. When you are satiated, stop eating.

4. Get moving.

Exercising can enhance your ketones when you are eating Ketotarian and/or fasting intermittently. One way to maximize this positive effect of exercise is to work out in the morning before you eat breakfast or while you are fasting. Research has shown that fasted workouts increase ketones more than exercising after a meal.[5]

5. Try coconut or MCT oil.

Having some coconut or MCT (medium-chain triglycerides) oil is one hack to help you get into ketosis. Coconut oil contains some MCT oil, and MCT oil is the pure source of these bioavailable fats.

MCT oil is easily absorbed for energy and an easy way to increase ketones.[6] These fats are so good at increasing ketosis that they can work even in the presence of higher carb intake.[7] Coconut oil also contains a specific MCT called lauric acid, which has been shown to create a more sustained ketosis.[8]

One word of advice for coconut and MCT oil: start off slowly. Too much of this stuff and your stomach can cramp and it can cause diarrhea. Start with 1 teaspoon per day and work your way up to 2 to 3 tablespoons a day.

6. Manage your stress.

Being chronically stressed is another reason I find that people have trouble getting into ketosis. Stress can cause hormone imbalances and higher inflammation levels. Not good for your metabolism. Check out the Ketotarian Toolbox in Chapter 7 for a full guide to dealing with this important factor to not only ketosis but your overall health.

7. Try intermittent fasting.

One of my favorite ways to boost ketosis is intermittent fasting (IF). This tool can be personalized to work for the individual. For a full guide on the different ways to fast intermittently, check out the Ketotarian Toolbox in Chapter 7.

what the heck is the keto flu and how can i avoid it?

For most of your life you have been living off of carbohydrates to fuel your body. Now that this is changing, so will your body. Every cell, tissue, and fiber of our being has relied on this one macronutrient (carbohydrates) for so long that when we switch to something else it can take some time to adjust, and some of us can go through a metabolic detoxing period or what is called the keto flu. Your brain and metabolism have to shift from burning the dirty sugar fuel to healthy clean fat fuel, and that can cause some detox symptoms for some people.

Our fat cells can also be a storage place for toxins like heavy metals and chemical hormone disruptors. When we first become a fat burner, this can cause the release of these stored toxins, another possible component to the keto flu for some people.

The metabolic shift into nutritional ketosis will also shift your gut microbiome (your bacteria eat what you eat). Someone with an underlying bacterial dysbiosis or yeast overgrowth can experience "die-off" symptoms from changing the foods they (and their bacteria) eat.

Increasing your carbohydrates will lower keto flu symptoms, but from a functional-medicine perspective, I am more interested in finding out what is contributing to these symptoms in the first place. Supporting detox pathways or microbiome health with herbal or botanical medicines may be appropriate for people dealing with these issues.

These symptoms can last anywhere from a couple of days to a couple of weeks and are similar to flu-like symptoms.

Common Keto Flu Symptoms

- Fatigue
- Headache
- Nausea
- Insomnia
- Irritability
- Upset stomach

Not everyone will experience these symptoms, and if you do, they may not be the same as for the next person. You may never even encounter any of these issues, or you may start off great and then experience mild symptoms after a couple of weeks in. So what are some things we can do to help prevent these symptoms and/or overcome them?

Overcoming the Keto Flu

- Drink more water (half of your body weight in ounces).
- Increase your healthy fat intake.
- Increase sea salt and mineral intake (electrolyte-rich foods). See the Ketotarian food list in Chapter 4 and the Ketotarian Toolbox in Chapter 7.
- Manage your stress. See the Ketotarian Toolbox in Chapter 7.
- Exercise

step 4.
give yourself an 8-week ketotarian reset

I suggest trying the Ketotarian plan in this book for at least 60 days, although I do include some optional modifications after 30 days in Chapter 7.

Through this (at least) 60-day journey, you will shift your body's metabolism to that of an efficient fat-burning state. After 8 weeks, reassess where you are and how you feel. If you are satisfied with where you are, you don't need to change anything. You are eating some of the most nutrient-dense foods on the planet. But does everyone need to stay in nutritional ketosis permanently? Absolutely not. In 8 weeks, you will find your groove. Experiment with the Ketotarian Tools in the next chapter, such as intermittent fasting and your personal carb tolerance. Spend varying times out of ketosis if you want by increasing your healthy carbs, lowering your healthy fats, and see how you feel.

When your body is metabolically agile from your time in ketosis, you can ebb and flow more effortlessly. This is grace-based eating instead of punishing your body with food through fad, crash dieting and insatiable cravings.

7

ketotarian toolbox:
**Intermittent Fasting and
Other Tips and Tricks**

ketotarian tool:
ketotarian intermittent fasting (IF)

In addition to all the healthy keto foods to focus on, another way to get yourself into a ketogenic, fat-adapted state is intermittent fasting (IF), or periods of calorie restriction. And because this is another way to become keto-adapted, it's also another tool to use to bring inflammation levels down. I personally use this tool on a regular basis and have seen it work for countless patients. Intermittent fasting has the health blogosphere all abuzz. Here's what you need to know.

Intermittent fasting is a general term for a period of time in which you limit food intake or don't eat at all. Why would anyone want to put themselves through periods of starvation? Well, studies have shown that IF could significantly bring down markers of inflammation. In fact, research is showing a few fascinating ways that intermittent fasting calms different types of inflammation and mTOR (a pro-cancer pathway) while increasing autophagy (cell cleaning and recycling) and the AMPK and Nrf2 pathways (disease-fighting pathways):

- **Brain inflammation.** Mental health problems like anxiety, depression, and brain fog are on the rise, and studies are showing that IF improves brain function and mood, having a sort of antidepressant effect. Neurological conditions like Alzheimer's disease and Parkinson's disease—as well as mood disorders such as depression and anxiety—are known as neuroinflammatory conditions, and IF looks promising for these as well. Other studies have shown that IF may actually protect neurons from genetic and epigenetic stress factors, meaning it can essentially slow down brain aging!

- **Lung inflammation.** Fasting every other day was shown to decrease asthma symptoms and markers of oxidative stress and inflammation.

- **Hormone-signaling inflammation.** Intermittent fasting decreases insulin resistance, a hormonal problem that affects a staggering 50 percent of American adults. It also increases production of beneficial enzymes that increase your body's ability to adapt to stress and fight chronic diseases like diabetes.

- **Chronic pain inflammation.** Intermittent fasting improves neuroplasticity—the ability of the brain to form and reorganize synaptic connections in response to new information—which researchers are studying for the role it may play in managing chronic pain.

- **Cancer.** Various studies have looked at the promising connection between intermittent fasting and reducing the risk of breast cancer.

- **Autoimmune conditions.** Fasting every three days has been shown to reduce symptoms of autoimmune conditions such as multiple sclerosis and lupus.

- **Gut inflammation.** In my practice, I've seen what a great tool IF can be for inflammatory bowel issues like stomach pain, IBS, colitis, diarrhea, and nausea. Research also reflects the benefits of fasting therapy for gut health.

- **Heart inflammation.** IF has been shown to reduce cardiovascular disease risk in part because of its ability to increase protective HDL cholesterol and reduce triglycerides and blood pressure.

- **Cravings and emotional eating.** Our culture is obsessed with food, and we eat all the time. As a result, most of us have lost touch with what it means to feel physical hunger. As my patients explore intermittent fasting, they learn more about their body and their emotional relationship with food. Through the different protocols of intermittent fasting, they often truly gain freedom from cravings and eating out of habit or for emotional reasons. Physically, consistent intermittent fasting transitions their metabolism from an erratic sugar-burning roller coaster to a slow and steady fat-burning machine.

WHAT ARE THE BEST METHODS OF INTERMITTENT FASTING?

Beginner

The 8-to-6 eating window

One simple way to IF is to try eating just from 8 a.m. to 6 p.m. This window allows for a longer fasting time that stretches from the early evening to a reasonable time in the morning.

The 12-to-6 eating window

This is the one I personally do during the workweek. It's the same as the last option, only this one extends the fasting period until lunchtime, when you'll have your first meal of the day. I drink lots of water and herbal tea in the morning and enjoy lunch so much more!

Intermediate

The modified 2-day plan

Another way to fast intermittently is to eat a regular clean diet for five days a week and then pick any two days of the week to restrict your intake of food to less than 700 calories. This caloric restriction still activates many of the same benefits as a full intermittent fasting day.

The 5-to-2 plan

Another simple intermittent fasting protocol is to completely fast for two whole non-consecutive days in a week—for example, fast on Monday and Wednesday but eat regular clean foods the other five days.

Advanced

The every-other-day plan

For this intermittent fasting protocol, you would fast fully every other day. This plan is a bit intense but can be great (and very effective) for some people.

Our culture is obsessed with food, and we eat all the time. As a result, most of us have lost touch with what it means to feel physical hunger.

BUT ISN'T INTERMITTENT FASTING HARMFUL FOR HORMONE HEALTH?

This is a question I get asked a lot. Let's look at the science on intermittent fasting and hormones.

Hunger and Fat Storing Hormones (Insulin, Ghrelin, and Leptin)

When it comes to improving the hormones that directly impact your hunger, blood sugar, and metabolism, this is where intermittent fasting shines. This is one of the top tools I use for blood sugar problems. Intermittent fasting has been shown to decrease insulin resistance, reducing diabetes risks[1] and enhancing metabolism.[2] Intermittent fasting has also been shown to have a positive effect on the hormone ghrelin. Surprisingly, the changes in ghrelin release during IF improved dopamine levels in the brain, improving cognitive function.[3] This is another example of the gut-brain axis at work in your body.

If your blood sugar is not stable, I suggest easing into intermittent fasting protocols slowly, working gently with your body as you create glucose stability.

Leptin resistance, another hormonal resistance pattern that can lead to stubborn weight gain, is another issue for which I use IF.

Female Hormones (Estrogen and Progesterone)

If you are female, the brain-ovary axis or hypothalamic-pituitary-gonadal (HPG) axis is your brain's communication with your ovaries. Your brain speaks by sending hormones, which are basically chemical emails, to the ovaries. This then prompts your ovaries to release estrogen and progesterone. A healthy HPG axis is essential for you to feel great and also for pregnancy.

Women tend to be more sensitive to intermittent fasting, due at least in part to something called kisspeptin. This little guy stimulates the hypothalamus to release the chemical email GnRH in both men and women. But women tend to have more kisspeptin. Research suggests that higher kisspeptin levels in women create a greater sensitivity to things like fasting.[4]

This can cause women who try intermittent fasting to miss their period, throw off their cycle, or just make them overall feel hormonally imbalanced and not as good.

This could, in theory, affect fertility as well as metabolism, although more studies need to be done.

But no two people are exactly alike. Clinically I find that some women do great with intermittent fasting and some don't. Does this mean that females who are sensitive to intermittent fasting shouldn't do it at all? Not entirely. For these individuals, it may just require a gentler approach. That's where crescendo fasting comes in.

Crescendo fasting is a tool I use for my patients who don't do well with other intermittent fasting.

Here's exactly how to do crescendo fasting:

1. Fast 2 nonconsecutive days a week (such as Monday and Friday).

2. On fasting days, take it easy on the exercise. Maybe light walking or gentle yoga.

3. Aim for a fast of 12 to 16 hours.

4. After 2 weeks, try adding another fasting day (such as Monday, Wednesday, and Friday).

5. During this protocol I typically suggest adding around 6 grams of branched chain amino acid supplements (BCAAs), which come in powder and capsule form. BCAAs help take the edge off and improve the experience and positive impact of the fast.

The beginner forms of intermittent fasting mentioned earlier can also be good options here.

Cortisol

Your main stress hormone, cortisol, is secreted by your adrenal glands, which sit on top of your kidneys like little hats. Adrenal fatigue, which I have written a lot about over the years, occurs when your brain-adrenal balance (hypothalamic-pituitary-adrenal [HPA] axis) is off kilter. Cortisol can be high when it should be low, low when it should be high, always high, or always low. In short, there are different variations of HPA axis dysfunction. In general, I find that people with circadian rhythm issues like this aren't rock stars with many kinds of intermittent fasting. If you have a circadian rhythm dysfunction but still want to experiment with IF, I suggest starting with the beginner options.

Thyroid Hormones (T4 and T3)

The queen of all hormones impacts every single cell of your awesomely designed body. If your thyroid isn't working well, nothing is. The crazy thing about thyroid hormone problems is that there are many different reasons for them.

There are autoimmune thyroid problems like Hashimoto's disease; thyroid conversion issues like low T3 syndrome; thyroid resistance, which is similar to insulin resistance; and thyroid problems that are secondary to brain-thyroid (hypothalamic-pituitary-thyroid, or HPT) axis dysfunction. Each of these thyroid hormone pathway disorders can respond differently to intermittent fasting. What I have found, however, is that while fasting can lower thyroid hormones, that is not necessarily a bad thing. Someone who intermittently fasts regularly and eats a healthy fat-based ketogenic diet can have slightly lower thyroid levels but still feel fantastic. This is just their body needing less of the hormone to function; similar to a hybrid car, it's more efficient with its energy. However, some people with thyroid problems don't do very well with fasting, making intermittent fasting a case-by-case tool for people with thyroid issues. It's all about context.

WHAT DO YOU EAT BETWEEN INTERMITTENT FASTING WINDOWS?

It's important to remember that you ultimately can't fast your way out of a bad diet. If you want to try out intermittent fasting for yourself, you will want to make sure your diet complements your intermittent fasting endeavors. When you are not fasting, focusing on the healthy fats, safe carbs, and clean protein in the Ketotarian plan is important if you want the full benefits of intermittent fasting.

Fasting-Mimicking Diet

Another tool, similar to intermittent fasting, that you can experiment with in your Ketotarian lifestyle is the Fasting Mimicking Diet (FMD). FMD is what its name implies: the benefits of fasting, without the fasting part; that is, another hack to promote nutritional ketosis and fat loss, boost the brain, enhance autophagy, and calm inflammation.

FMD is the evolution of decades of pioneering work by Dr. Valter Longo and his team at the University of South California. It is centered on caloric restriction for a period of time. Here's what FMD looks like:

- **Day 1:** Eat 1,100 calories.

- **Days 2–5:** Eat 800 calories per day.

For these five days, your macronutrients should look like this:

- **80 percent fat**

- **10 percent protein**

- **10 percent carbohydrate**

During the five days of calorie restriction, do not exercise, and limit your coffee to a max of 1 cup a day. The great thing is that the research on FMD used many of same foods in the Ketotarian plan—healthy plant fats.[5] Fasting mimicking diets, like intermittent fasting, is a way to increase ketosis and all its health benefits such as autophagy and lowering inflammation. If you are nursing or pregnant, this is not a time for calorie restriction, but most other people can benefit from these fasting and caloric restriction protocols.

ketotarian tool: find your carb sweet spot

This tool can be used once you have done your Ketotarian plan for at least 1 month (but preferably at least 60 days—I'm being flexible here since we are all different). This means you have eaten your high amounts of healthy fats and kept your healthy carbohydrates to 55 grams net carbs or less. This will give your body some time to switch from being a sugar-burner to a fat-burner (keto-adapted).

If you feel great on this macronutrient ratio, there is no reason whatsoever to use the Carb Sweet Spot tool. Since we are all different, some people, once they are fat-adapted, find they feel better with slightly higher carb levels. This tool is a great way to find out where you do the best with carbohydrates.

After at least one month of having your carbohydrates at less than 55 grams net carbs, you can do the following:

1. Moderate your carbs.

Increase your carbs to 75 to 155 grams net carbs every day and reduce your healthy fat intake to compensate for this increase (example: 20% carbs, 65% fat, 15% protein). For example, try adding in some of these healthy carb options with your non-starchy vegetables that you have already been eating, such as more fruit or starchy vegetables. Some examples:

- cooked carrots (8 grams net carbs per 1 cup)
- blueberries (18 grams net carbs per 1 cup)
- other fruits
- baked sweet potato (23 grams net carbs per potato)
- baked yam (33 grams net carbs per yam)

Some women do well with this slightly higher level of carbs, and there's nothing wrong with it. There should be no shame in eating more of these healthy carbs if this is where you feel the best. If you are going to increase your carbs to these levels, I suggest having them around dinnertime, to avoid throwing off your metabolism during the day. By having your carbs in the evening, you also can capitalize on their fatiguing effect to help you wind down before bed. Some people do well by increasing their carbs before or after a heavy workout. I suggest testing your ketones through this self-experimentation to further understand the effects on your system.

2. Cycle your carbs.

Continue to eat your normal Ketotarian high-fat, low-carbohydrate diet (less than 55 grams net carbs per day) for 5 to 6 days a week; then increase your carbs to 75 to 155 grams net carbs on the 6th and 7th day(s) using the above healthy carb list (example: 20% carbs, 65% fat, 15% protein). This cyclical Ketotarian approach can be a good approach for some people, particularly women and endurance athletes, and it's a good option if you are at a weight-loss plateau for more than a month. This is a tool to further personalize your Ketotarian experience.

Generally, I do not suggest increasing carbohydrates to the higher end of this range for people who tend to have carb sensitivities such as those with insulin resistance, diabetes, or inflammatory issues or those who have more than 10 pounds of weight to lose. And to reiterate, no one needs to increase their carbohydrates if they feel great.

If you decide you want to test these two Carb Sweet Spot tools, try each separately for a month and see how you feel. Compare your energy levels, brain function, weight, mood, sleep, and digestion. Where do you feel the best?

3. Seasonal ketotarian

Another tool you can consider once you have done the Ketotarian plan for at least 60 days is to go into ketosis seasonally. From an ancestral health perspective, this tool mimics the cycles that humans would have done throughout history. During the winter months, when fruit was scarce, our ancestors would naturally eat fewer carbohydrates. During the summer, however, they would graze on more berries and starchy tubers such as sweet potatoes. I have seen this tool of adjusting your foods with the seasons work wonderfully for those who have the metabolic flexibility to tolerate higher carbohydrates from real foods.

So, which tool should you use after 60 days? What makes Ketotarianism so sustainable is that it is centered around balance and finding your own. Experiment and have fun with it. After 60 days following the guidelines in this book, play around with these foods. Should you stay in ketosis long term? Many people who are prone to insulin or weight-loss resistance, insatiable cravings, or neurological problems thrive in longer-term nutritional ketosis. Others do great with moderating their carbs seasonally or throughout the week as outlined above.

Some people even do well with higher carbs from real foods, but love to go back to ketosis when they want a metabolic reset. Remember, this is about grace and lightness, not dieting dogma and shame.

Find out what your body loves and hates by using the tools in this book.

ketotarian tool: electrolyte balance

When you have gone Ketotarian and cut out all the inflammatory carbohydrates like grains and sugar, your body will lose fluid retention. For some, this can also throw off electrolyte balance (specifically, sodium, potassium, and magnesium) during this metabolic transition. You can replenish those electrolytes by adding sea salt into your diet. Some of my patients who have HPA axis issues or what's commonly referred to as "adrenal fatigue" have 1 teaspoon of Himalayan sea salt in a glass of water in the morning or add it to their meals. You can also dissolve 1 to 2 vegetable or chicken bone broth bouillon cubes or 1 to 2 teaspoons of sea salt in a cup of water. Focusing on some of my favorite Ketotarian foods like avocado, mushrooms, and spinach will also provide you with potassium and magnesium, which will balance this issue. In addition to foods, there are also some great electrolyte supplements on the market.

ketotarian tool: manage your stress

Stress is one of the hidden reasons why some people have a difficult time getting into ketosis.

Stress is also associated with a lot of conditions including a greater risk of depression, anxiety, heart disease, gastrointestinal problems, and autoimmune conditions. In fact, studies have found that workplace stress is as detrimental to your health as secondhand smoke.[6] And psychological stress actually weakens your immune system and increases inflammation in the body.

Here are my suggestions to start moving beyond repetitive thoughts and manage stress to maximize your physical health:

* **Set your alarm earlier.**
  - The seed of the day is the morning—so start it off right. Instead of hitting the snooze button one too many times, give yourself plenty of time to slowly wake up. Have a glass of green tea and spend time in silence, centering yourself for the day. Running around the house at the last minute because you slept in sets off a stressful start to the day.

- **Practice awareness.**
  - Awareness is like a muscle—you have to use it to make it stronger. Tools like mindfulness meditation will help you grow in awareness. You'll come to see that you're not your thoughts but the observer of them. That breaks the repetitive mind chatter and brings you into the present moment.

- **Write a reasonable to-do list.**
  - I recommend getting to work a little early—that may sound horrible to some, but it will give you time to yourself to focus your day.
  - Take a few minutes out of your morning to make a list of what you would like to accomplish. Start with more pressing needs, and then work your way to longer-term goals. Highlight the tasks as they are accomplished.
  - This approach will gather the mental clutter and organize it all into an orderly list. But also remember, if it all doesn't get done today, give yourself grace— there is always tomorrow.

- **Try a tech detox.**
  - The Internet has allowed us to have quality, helpful information at our fingertips. But while it's one thing to use it to grow in awareness, it's another thing to mindlessly scroll through status updates as mind-numbing hours pass you by. This is often a way for you to avoid the present moment, and it prevents you from moving beyond repetitive thought. Turn down the chatter and unplug.

- **Focus on each task, one by one.**
  - As you are moving through the day's to-do list, remain present with the task at hand. Preoccupied thoughts about the future or the past can cause anxiety and decrease your effectiveness.
  - Don't make boring work a means to an end, simply watching the clock tick by. However mundane your to-do list may be, honor it. Let that present moment be a meditation exercise. Fully accepting the task decreases stress and can help bring you inner peace.

- **Organize your space mindfully.**
  - Clutter on the outside can cause clutter on the inside. Schedule time each week to clean up your desk and office space. Throw away papers and items that you don't need. Minimizing office and home mess is a great way to bring calm to your day.

- **Try tai chi or yoga.**
  - After you turn down the mental and social media chatter, fill the time gaps with exercises of silence. Tai chi and yoga are two great ways to grow in inner stillness.

- **Practice conscious breathing throughout the day.**
  - When we're stressed and holding in tension, our breath can become shallow—which only feeds the anxiety further. Observing your breath is a fundamental way to bring inner stillness to your day.
  - I recommend conscious breathing to anchor you in the present moment. Whenever you find yourself getting stressed at work, take a few moments to just breathe naturally and focus on those breaths, letting worries and anxieties diffuse and drift away.

- **Fill your mind with positivity.**
  - Negative and stressful thoughts can be softened by reading or listening to positive things. For example, classical or meditation music, a happy podcast, a self-help book, or just silence can be the perfect path to quieting the mind. Research confirms that we can rewire our brain the more we do something—so make positivity a habit.

- **Surround yourself with positive people.**
  - The people you spend most of your time with will either build you up or feed into negative thoughts. I like to imagine the three circles of friendship: the first should be your inner circle of friends who mutually lift each other up. The next circle should be people you can be a positive influence on. The last, outer circle is anyone who will negatively influence you. Keep your distance

from these "energy vampires," who are constantly negative or make every conversation about themselves. Love them from a healthy distance.

- **Don't be offended.**
  - I've met many patients who are blanketed with pain from years of being offended, so much so that it's affecting their health. Replaying a negative event repeatedly in your mind can negatively impact your body. No matter how justified you may be, consider making forgiveness part of your healing. Realize that whatever was done to you was not personal but was the unconsciousness in the other person. Easier said than done, I understand, but not taking things personally is liberating—and good for your health.

- **Head outside at least once during the day.**
  - When you have a break, go soak up some sun. Vitamin D, the sunshine vitamin, is essential for lifting your mood and brain function. If it's not a sunny day, simply going outside can still take the edge off a stressful workday.
  - Find a way to connect with nature. Even if there's just one tree outside your office, go sit next to that tree! Sit still for a moment and practice your conscious breathing.

- **Get quality sleep.**
  - Be sure to get enough zzz's at night to ensure that you're recharged for the next day. Optimal sleep for most people is around seven hours per night. Turning off the TV and cell phone before bed and reading a book instead is one simple way to promote quality sleep.

ketotarian tool:
make peace with food and your body

This tool is not directly measurable like finding your carb tolerance, intermittent fasting, electrolyte balancing, and even managing your stress, but it is essential nonetheless. You can get your macronutrients perfect, eat the healthiest foods, and become a perfect fat-burning, keto-adapted machine, but in my experience, if your relationship with food and your body is unhealthy, you are not going to enjoy all the goodness a Ketotarian lifestyle has to offer.

In my years of clinical experience, Ketotarianism (or any way of healthy eating, for that matter) is at its best when it's born out of a healthy relationship with food. Make food your friend. Focus on all the nutrient-dense filling foods that make your body thrive. The key is to eat them consciously and rationally.

—

Eating with awareness brings a lightness and grace to food, your body, and life.

—

Eliminating the foods we are avoiding is not a way to punish your body but to focus instead on foods that your body loves. Your body is a gift that has taken care of you. Love yourself enough to nourish your body with good food medicine.

Your body is alive because of brilliant biochemistry. With each meal, focus on how you can fuel yourself. If you decide to try intermittent fasting, do it because you love your body—and because you are eating satiating foods around your fast, you can do intermittent fasting with ease.

Eating with awareness brings a lightness and grace to food, your body, and life. This grace-based eating paired with the natural fat-adapted curbing of cravings are the two magical ingredients of true food freedom.

You can't heal a body you hate. Forgiving yourself and others can be a revolutionary act of healing. I consider this emotional healing to be vital in my work helping patients overcome their health obstacles.

Research estimates that a staggering 90 percent of our thoughts are repetitive. For many people, these thoughts are not just repetitive, they're also negative. This chronic stress can raise inflammation in our bodies and can contribute to health problems in the long term—unless it's kept in check.

Further, research found that we make about two hundred food-related decisions each day. The problem is that most of these food decisions, the researchers found, were made on mindless autopilot. We aren't consciously aware we're making most of them, which could be further contributing to poor eating habits.

That's why increased consciousness of our thoughts is the first step to healing and long-term health. Observing the presence of our thoughts brings us into the here and now and breaks the addictive cycle of our past.

I recommend practicing mindfulness meditation as one way to become more aware of our health choices and eliminate negative, repetitive thought patterns so that we can become more fully present, in tune with our bodies, and able to achieve optimum health.

Out of mindful awareness of who you were created to be, your intrinsic worth, will flow healthy choices. Self-care is a form of self-respect. If you recognize that you are a Tesla instead of an old used car, how would that impact how you treat your body, mind, and spirit? True, sustainable wellness is not about shame or rules, it's about loving yourself enough to nourish your body with rest, movement, and delicious food medicine.

ketotarian manifested:
The Recipes + Meal Plans

From manifesto to manifested. Now that we have gone over all the important reasons to go Ketotarian, let's put this delicious, healing food medicine into action. The Ketotarian recipes all have keys for your convenience: vegan, vegetarian, and AIP (autoimmune protocol or autoimmune friendly). All recipes are gluten-free, grain-free, dairy-free (except ghee), and paleo friendly. Macronutrients are listed per serving for each recipe.

8

veggie main dishes

This is the foundation of your Ketotarian journey: fresh, clean plant foods, done the right way. You don't have to eat like a rabbit, munching on kale all day, to be healthy (no offense, kale; I love you). Fill up and fuel yourself with decadent healthy-plant-fat foods. Use the recipes in this section as delicious food medicine to nourish your cells and feed your gut microbiome. Instead of doing another detox, make your life a cleanse with the vegan and vegetarian ketogenic foods in this section.

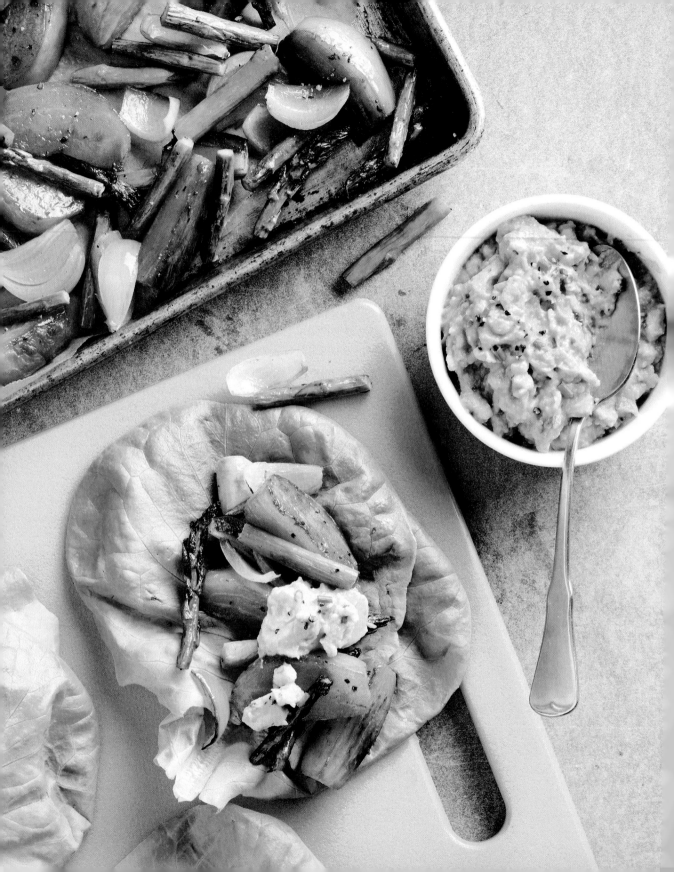

spring veggie lettuce wraps

VEGAN, VEGETARIAN, AIP

PREP: 15 minutes
ROAST: 45 minutes

SERVES 2

2 medium orange or yellow beets (about 3 inches in diameter), peeled and cut into ½-inch-thick wedges

3 tablespoons olive oil

½ teaspoon coarse salt

¼ teaspoon freshly ground black pepper

1 small shallot, cut into thin wedges

8 ounces fresh asparagus, trimmed and cut into 1-inch pieces

1 large avocado, halved, pitted, and peeled

2 tablespoons fresh lime juice

1 tablespoon chopped fresh chives

8 large Bibb lettuce leaves

1 Preheat the oven to 425°F. In a shallow baking pan, toss together the beet wedges, 1½ tablespoons oil, ¼ teaspoon salt, and ⅛ teaspoon pepper. Spread the mixture in a single layer in the pan. Cover the pan with foil. Roast for 30 minutes. Uncover, add the shallot wedges, and roast, uncovered, for 10 minutes more. Add the asparagus and drizzle with the remaining 1½ teaspoons oil. Roast, uncovered, for 8 to 10 minutes more, or until the vegetables are tender and starting to turn brown.

2 Meanwhile, in a medium bowl combine the avocado, juice, chives, the remaining ¼ teaspoon salt, and the remaining ⅛ teaspoon pepper. Mash to the desired consistency using a potato masher or fork.

3 To serve, stack the lettuce leaves to make four stacks of two leaves each. Spoon the roasted vegetables on top of the lettuce stacks. Spoon the avocado mixture evenly over the vegetables. Wrap the lettuce around the vegetables and avocado mixture and serve.

Protein: 3 g • **Net Carbs:** 11 g • **Fat:** 32 g

thai vegetable cashew curry with coconut

VEGAN, VEGETARIAN

PREP: 10 minutes
COOK: 35 minutes

SERVES 2

¼ cup coconut oil

¼ cup chopped red onion

2 teaspoons minced fresh garlic

2 teaspoons minced fresh ginger

3 tablespoons sugar-free Thai red or green curry paste

1 large yellow or red bell pepper, cut into 1-inch dice

¼ teaspoon sea salt

2 Japanese eggplants, cut into 1-inch dice

1 cup full-fat coconut milk

2 teaspoons fresh lime juice

½ cup raw unsalted cashews, lightly toasted and coarsely chopped

3 tablespoons shredded unsweetened coconut, very lightly toasted

½ teaspoon fresh lime zest

1 Heat the oil in a 12-inch skillet over medium-high heat. When hot, add the onion, garlic, and ginger and sauté until the onion is translucent, about 4 minutes. Stir in the curry paste and cook for 1 minute.

2 Add the bell pepper and salt and sauté until halfway tender, about 5 minutes. Add the eggplants and sauté for 3 minutes. Cover the pan and reduce the heat to medium-low. Cook until the eggplants and bell pepper are fully tender, about 10 minutes.

3 Uncover the pan and stir in the milk and juice. Bring to a boil over high heat. Boil until the sauce thickens slightly, about 4 minutes. Ladle between two bowls, sprinkling with the nuts, coconut, and zest.

Protein: 11 g • **Net Carbs:** 29 g • **Fat:** 62 g

mushroom–red wine ragout with brussels sprouts, olives, and herbs

VEGAN, VEGETARIAN

PREP: 20 minutes
COOK: 20 minutes

SERVES 2

¼ cup olive oil

½ cup finely chopped red onion

2 teaspoons minced fresh garlic

1 tablespoon tomato paste

½ pound white button mushrooms, ends trimmed, quartered

½ pound medium Brussels sprouts, ends trimmed, quartered

1 teaspoon herbes de Provence

¼ teaspoon sea salt

⅛ teaspoon ground white pepper

12 pitted kalamata olives, halved

¼ cup dry red wine

½ cup preservative-free, sugar-free vegetable broth or stock

1 Heat 2 tablespoons of the oil in a 10-inch skillet over medium-high heat. Once hot, add the onion and garlic and sauté until the onion is translucent, about 4 minutes. Add the tomato paste and sauté for 1 minute.

2 Add the remaining 2 tablespoons oil to the pan. Add the mushrooms, Brussels sprouts, herbes de Provence, salt, and pepper and sauté until the vegetables are tender and the liquid has cooked off, 5 to 7 minutes. Add the olives and sauté for 1 minute.

3 Add the wine and bring to a boil over high heat. Boil for 1 minute. Add the broth and boil until the liquid is thickened and reduced by half, 5 to 7 minutes.

Protein: 8 g • Net Carbs: 15 g • Fat: 33 g

spaghetti squash with pine nuts and basil

VEGETARIAN

PREP: 15 minutes

ROAST: 40 minutes

COOL: 5 minutes

SERVES 2

One 1½- to 2-pound spaghetti squash

⅓ cup pine nuts

½ cup loosely packed dried dulse

2 tablespoons olive oil

2 green onions (scallions)

1 cup chopped, peeled eggplant

½ cup chopped red bell pepper

1 garlic clove, minced

2 tablespoons fresh lemon juice

2 tablespoons dry white wine

2 tablespoons ghee

¼ cup chopped fresh basil leaves

¼ teaspoon coarse salt

¼ teaspoon freshly ground black pepper

½ cup pitted green or kalamata olives, chopped

1 Preheat the oven to 400°F. Line a medium baking sheet with parchment paper or foil. Cut the spaghetti squash in half crosswise. Use a spoon to scrape out the seeds and strings. Place the squash halves, cut side down, on the prepared pan. Roast for 40 to 50 minutes, or until just tender (a thin sharp knife should be able to easily pierce the squash). Cool slightly on a wire rack.

2 Meanwhile, in a medium skillet cook the pine nuts over medium-low heat, stirring frequently, for 3 to 5 minutes, or until lightly toasted. Immediately transfer the nuts to a small bowl; set aside. Add the dulse and 1 tablespoon of the oil to the same skillet. Cook over medium heat for 3 to 5 minutes, or until the dulse is lightly browned, stirring occasionally. Transfer the dulse to a plate; set aside.

3 Thinly slice the green onions, keeping the white and green parts separate. Add the white parts to the same skillet. Add the remaining 1 tablespoon oil and the eggplant, bell pepper, and garlic to the skillet. Cook over medium heat, stirring occasionally, for 3 to 5 minutes, or until the vegetables are crisp-tender. Transfer the vegetables to a large bowl; cover to keep warm.

<u>4</u> Add the juice and wine to the skillet; cook and stir over medium heat until boiling, scraping up any browned bits from the bottom of the skillet. Reduce the heat to medium-low. Add 1 tablespoon ghee; cook and whisk until completely melted and combined. Repeat with the remaining 1 tablespoon ghee. Remove from the heat.

<u>5</u> Using a pot holder, hold one half of the squash in one hand. Using a fork, separate the squash strands and scrape into the bowl with the eggplant mixture. Repeat with the remaining squash half. Toss the squash and vegetables to combine. Add the pine nuts, 2 tablespoons basil, and the salt and black pepper. Toss to combine. Divide the squash mixture between two serving plates. Drizzle evenly with the sauce from the skillet. Top with the olives and green onions and the remaining 2 tablespoons basil. Crumble the dulse over each serving.

Protein: 7 g • **Net Carbs:** 21 g • **Fat:** 58 g

moroccan vegetable tagine with olives and cinnamon-ghee almonds

VEGETARIAN

PREP: 20 minutes
COOK: 20 minutes

SERVES 2

¼ cup plus 1 tablespoon ghee

2 yellow, orange, or red bell peppers, cut into small dice

1 small red onion, cut into small dice

1 teaspoon minced fresh garlic

1 teaspoon minced fresh ginger

⅜ teaspoon sea salt

⅛ teaspoon plus a dash of ground cinnamon

⅛ teaspoon ground cumin

Dash of cayenne pepper

1 tablespoon tomato paste

1 small zucchini, cut into small dice

1½ cups packed fresh Swiss chard leaves, thinly sliced

1 cup preservative-free, sugar-free vegetable broth or stock

¼ cup pitted green olives, halved

½ cup raw unsalted almonds, coarsely chopped

2 tablespoons finely chopped fresh cilantro or parsley leaves

1 Heat 2 tablespoons of the ghee in a deep 10-inch skillet over medium-high heat. When hot, add the bell peppers, onion, garlic, ginger, ¼ teaspoon salt, ⅛ teaspoon cinnamon, and the cumin and cayenne and sauté until the onion is translucent, about 4 minutes. Stir in the tomato paste and cook for 1 minute.

2 Add the zucchini and sauté until tender, about 5 minutes. Stir in the chard and sauté until the chard is wilted, about 3 minutes. Add the broth and olives and bring to a boil over high heat. Once the mixture comes to a boil, cover the pan and reduce the heat to medium-low. Simmer until all of the vegetables are tender and the sauce thickens slightly, 10 to 15 minutes. Stir in 2 tablespoons ghee and let it melt.

3 While the tagine cooks, heat the remaining 1 tablespoon ghee in a small skillet over medium heat. Once melted, add the almonds and the remaining ⅛ teaspoon salt and a dash of cinnamon. Toast the almonds until light golden brown, about 3 minutes (do not let them burn).

4 Ladle the tagine between two large bowls and sprinkle each portion with the almonds and cilantro.

Protein: 12 g • **Net Carbs:** 21 g • **Fat:** 51 g

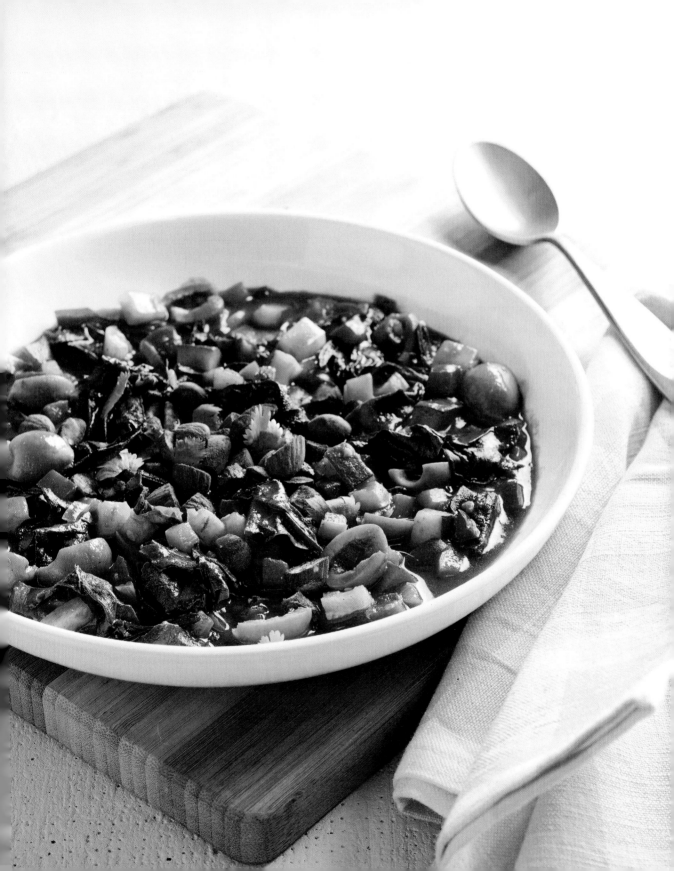

meatless mexican kale enchiladas

VEGAN, VEGETARIAN

PREP: 15 minutes
COOK: 30 minutes

SERVES 2

1 cup peeled, diced rutabaga

2 tablespoons avocado oil

⅔ cup chopped walnuts

½ cup chopped onion

¼ cup diced orange or yellow bell pepper

½ cup diced, seeded poblano pepper

3 garlic cloves, minced

1 teaspoon paprika

¾ teaspoon coarse salt

½ teaspoon dried oregano

½ teaspoon ground cumin

⅜ teaspoon freshly ground black pepper

¼ cup tomato paste

6 large lacinato kale leaves, stems trimmed*

6 tablespoons soft fresh vegan cheese, crumbled

1 Preheat the oven to 425°F. In a 2-quart rectangular baking dish toss together the rutabaga and 1 tablespoon of the oil. Roast uncovered, stirring once or twice, for 15 to 20 minutes or until the rutabaga is just tender; remove the pan from the oven and reserve.

2 Meanwhile, in a dry medium skillet, toast the walnuts over medium-low heat until lightly browned, stirring frequently. Remove the nuts from the skillet; set aside. In the same skillet cook the onion, bell pepper, poblano pepper, and 2 garlic cloves in the remaining 1 tablespoon oil over medium heat, stirring occasionally, for 4 to 5 minutes, or until the vegetables are tender. Stir in the paprika, ½ teaspoon salt, oregano, cumin, and ¼ teaspoon black pepper. Stir together ½ cup water and the tomato paste. Add to the vegetables and bring to a boil. Reduce the heat to medium-low and simmer, covered, for 5 minutes, stirring occasionally. Remove from the heat. Stir in the rutabaga and walnuts.

3 Lay the kale leaves on a flat work surface. Evenly spoon the rutabaga mixture onto one end of the kale leaves. Sprinkle the cheese over the filling. Roll up the kale leaves over the filling. Place the filled kale leaves, seam sides down, in the baking dish used to roast the rutabaga.

1 large avocado, halved, pitted, and peeled

1 to 2 tablespoons fresh lime juice

Fresh salsa

Chopped fresh cilantro

4 Bake, covered, for 10 to 15 minutes or until heated through. Meanwhile, in a medium bowl combine the avocado, juice, the remaining garlic clove, the remaining 1/4 teaspoon salt, and the remaining 1/8 teaspoon pepper. Mash to the desired consistency with a potato masher or fork. To serve, transfer the kale enchiladas to two serving plates. Top with the mashed avocado, salsa, and cilantro.

Protein: 20 g · **Net Carbs:** 34 g · **Fat:** 72 g

*NOTE: Use a long thin knife to trim the stem so that it's even with the top of the leaf. It will make it easier to roll up.

italian cauliflower rice soup

VEGAN, VEGETARIAN

PREP: 5 minutes
COOK: 18 minutes

SERVES 3 TO 4

¼ cup plus 2 tablespoons olive oil

1 cup chopped white onion

1 cup red bell pepper, cut into bite-size strips

2 cups fresh riced cauliflower

2 garlic cloves, minced

1 teaspoon Italian seasoning

½ teaspoon salt

¼ teaspoon red pepper flakes

3 cups preservative-free, sugar-free vegetable broth or stock

1 can (14.5 ounces) diced tomatoes, undrained

2 cups fresh baby spinach leaves

4 ounces soft fresh vegan cheese, crumbled

¼ cup pitted black or green olives, quartered

2 tablespoons olive oil

1 In a large saucepan, heat ¼ cup of the oil over medium heat. Add the onion and bell pepper; cook for 3 minutes. Stir in the cauliflower, garlic, Italian seasoning, salt, and red pepper flakes; cook for 5 minutes, stirring occasionally.

2 Add the broth and tomatoes; bring to a boil. Reduce the heat to medium-low and simmer, uncovered, for 10 minutes. Remove from the heat; stir in the spinach.

3 Ladle the soup into serving bowls. Top with the cheese and olives. Drizzle with the remaining 2 tablespoons olive oil.

Protein: 4 g • **Net Carbs:** 16 g • **Fat:** 33 g

asian cabbage-mushroom soup

VEGAN, VEGETARIAN, AIP

PREP: 20 minutes
COOK: 15 minutes

SERVES 2

1 ounce dried shiitake
mushrooms

¾ cup boiling water

2 green onions (scallions), thinly
sliced (keep white and green
parts separate)

1½ cups fresh shiitake
mushrooms, stemmed and thinly
sliced, or thinly sliced button
mushrooms

1 small celery stalk, thinly sliced

3 tablespoons toasted
sesame oil

1 tablespoon finely chopped
fresh ginger

½ ounce dried arame sea
vegetables, crumbled

1 cup snap peas, trimmed and
cut in half diagonally

2 cups finely shredded bok choy

2 to 3 teaspoons coconut
aminos

½ cup full-fat coconut milk

2 tablespoons snipped fresh
cilantro

1 In a small bowl, combine the dried mushrooms
and boiling water; cover and let stand for
15 minutes. Strain the mushrooms through a
fine sieve, reserving the soaking water. Rinse
the strained mushrooms; coarsely chop the
mushrooms and add them back to the soaking
water.

2 In a large saucepan, cook the white parts of
the green onions, the fresh mushrooms, and the
celery in the sesame oil over medium-high heat,
stirring occasionally, for 5 to 6 minutes, or until
the vegetables are tender and lightly browned.

3 Add 3 cups water and the ginger, arame, and
rehydrated mushrooms with their soaking water.
Bring to a boil. Reduce the heat to low and
simmer, covered, for 5 minutes. Add the snap
peas; cook, covered, for 2 minutes. Add the bok
choy. Cook, covered, for 1 minute more. Remove
from the heat. Stir in the coconut aminos and
coconut milk. Ladle into shallow bowls to serve.
Top with the green onions and cilantro.

Protein: 7 g • **Net Carbs:** 18 g • **Fat:** 29 g

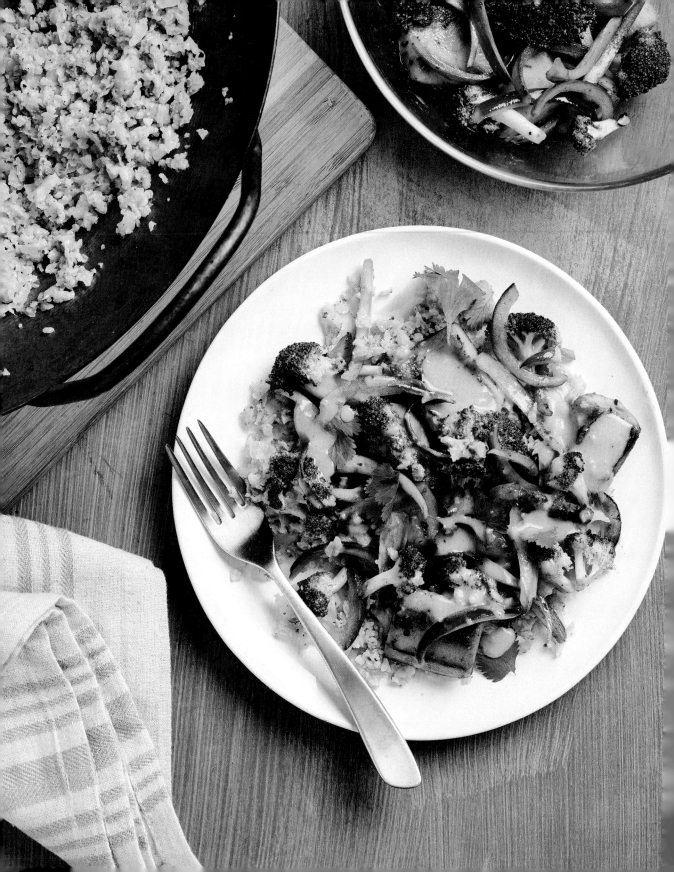

coconut veggie stir-fry with cauliflower rice

VEGAN, VEGETARIAN

PREP: 10 minutes
COOK: 15 minutes

SERVES 2

3 cups fresh cauliflower florets*

2 cups fresh broccoli florets

5 small pattypan squash, trimmed and quartered

2 tablespoons toasted sesame oil

⅓ cup thin slivers red onion

2 teaspoons grated fresh ginger

1 garlic clove, minced

¾ cup full-fat coconut milk

1 tablespoon liquid aminos

1 tablespoon cider vinegar

½ teaspoon coarse salt

¼ teaspoon freshly ground black pepper

2 tablespoons refined coconut oil

¼ cup unsweetened large coconut flakes, toasted

2 tablespoons snipped fresh cilantro

1 Place the cauliflower in the container of a food processor. Cover and pulse until the cauliflower is finely chopped (about the size of rice). Set aside.

2 In a large wok, stir-fry the broccoli and squash in the sesame oil over medium-high heat for 4 to 5 minutes, or until the vegetables are crisp-tender. Reduce the heat to medium if the vegetables brown too quickly. Add the onion and stir-fry for 2 minutes more. Transfer the vegetables to a bowl; cover to keep warm.

3 To the same wok, add the ginger and garlic. Cook and stir over medium-low heat for 30 seconds. Carefully add the coconut milk, liquid aminos, vinegar, ¼ teaspoon salt, and ⅛ teaspoon pepper. Bring to a boil. Reduce the heat to low and simmer, uncovered, for 5 minutes, or until the sauce is slightly thickened.

4 Meanwhile, in a large skillet heat the coconut oil over medium heat. Add the cauliflower rice, the remaining ¼ teaspoon salt, and the remaining ⅛ teaspoon pepper. Cook, stirring frequently, for 3 to 5 minutes, or until the cauliflower is just tender and starting to brown.

recipe continues

*TIP: If desired, substitute
3 cups purchased cauliflower
rice for the cauliflower florets.

<u>5</u> Return the vegetables to the wok. Cook and stir for 1 minute to heat through. Spoon the cauliflower rice evenly onto two serving plates. Top with the broccoli mixture and sauce. Sprinkle with the coconut and cilantro.

Protein: 9 g · **Net Carbs:** 15 g · **Fat:** 44 g

stuffed zucchini

VEGAN, VEGETARIAN

PREP: 20 minutes
BAKE: 30 minutes

SERVES 2

2 medium zucchini

3 tablespoons olive oil

¼ cup chopped yellow onion

1 garlic clove, minced

3 cups fresh baby spinach leaves

Salt and freshly ground black pepper

¼ cup soft fresh vegan cheese

¼ cup pitted black or green olives, coarsely chopped

1 teaspoon chopped fresh flat-leaf parsley

1 Preheat the oven to 375°F.

2 Cut the zucchini in half lengthwise; scoop out the pulp, leaving a ¼-inch shell. Chop the zucchini pulp.

3 In a large skillet, heat 2 tablespoons oil over medium heat. Add the zucchini pulp, onion, and garlic; cook for 3 to 5 minutes, until tender. Stir in the spinach; cook for 1 minute, or until wilted. Season with salt and pepper to taste. Remove from the heat; add the cheese and stir to combine. Spoon the spinach mixture into the zucchini shells. Place in a baking dish.

4 Bake, covered, for 20 minutes. Uncover and bake for 5 to 10 minutes more, or until the zucchini is just tender.

5 Meanwhile, in a small bowl, combine the olives, the parsley, and remaining 1 tablespoon oil. Spoon the olive mixture over the baked zucchini.

Protein: 6 g • **Net Carbs:** 8g • **Fat:** 26 g

zucchini and mushroom satay

VEGAN, VEGETARIAN

PREP: 15 minutes
COOK: 15 minutes

SERVES 2

½ yellow squash, cut into
1-inch pieces

½ zucchini, cut into 1-inch pieces

3 ounces shiitake mushrooms,
stems removed

FOR THE BASTE

2 tablespoons olive oil

1 teaspoon toasted sesame oil

1 teaspoon fresh lemon juice

½ teaspoon ground cumin

½ teaspoon ground coriander

½ teaspoon grated fresh ginger

1 garlic clove, minced

FOR THE ALMOND SAUCE

¼ cup finely chopped red onion

2 tablespoons full-fat coconut milk

2 tablespoons almond butter

2 tablespoons crushed almonds

¼ teaspoon cumin seeds

¼ teaspoon coriander seeds

¼ teaspoon sea salt

⅛ teaspoon cayenne pepper

1 garlic clove, finely minced

1 Preheat the broiler to high and position the upper rack 6 inches below the broiler. Prepare two 10-to-12-inch skewers; if using bamboo skewers, soak them in water for at least 30 minutes.

2 Skewer the squash and mushrooms evenly on the skewers. Place the skewers on the broiler pan.

3 Whisk together all of the baste ingredients. Brush half of the baste over the squash and mushrooms. Broil the skewers for 12 to 18 minutes, turning and brushing with the remaining baste several times.

4 Meanwhile, in a small saucepan, combine all of the almond sauce ingredients. Bring to a simmer over low heat and cook, stirring frequently, until thickened, about 3 to 4 minutes. Transfer to a bowl and serve with the finished skewers.

Protein: 7 g • **Net Carbs:** 8 g • **Fat:** 30 g

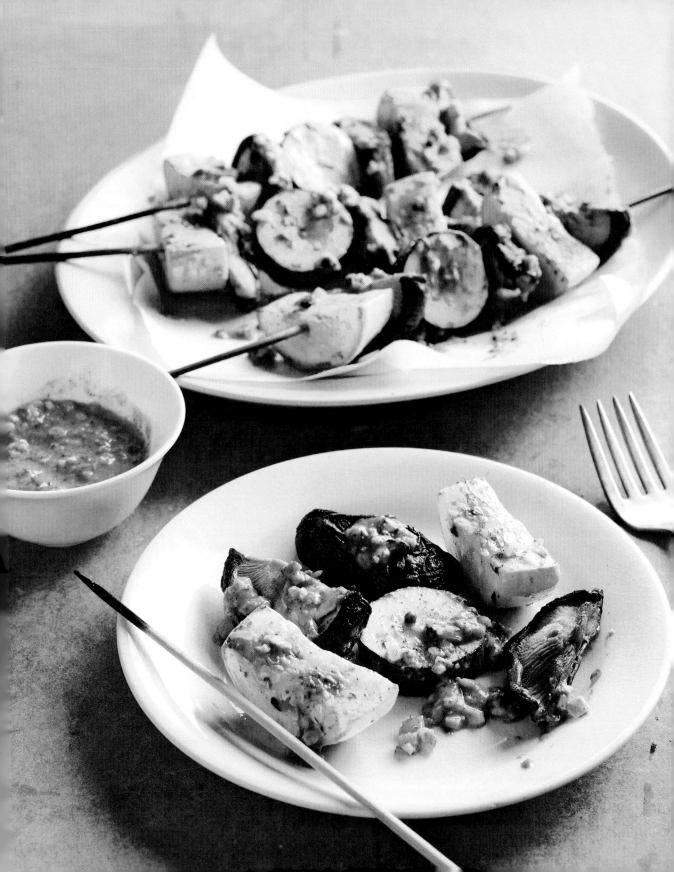

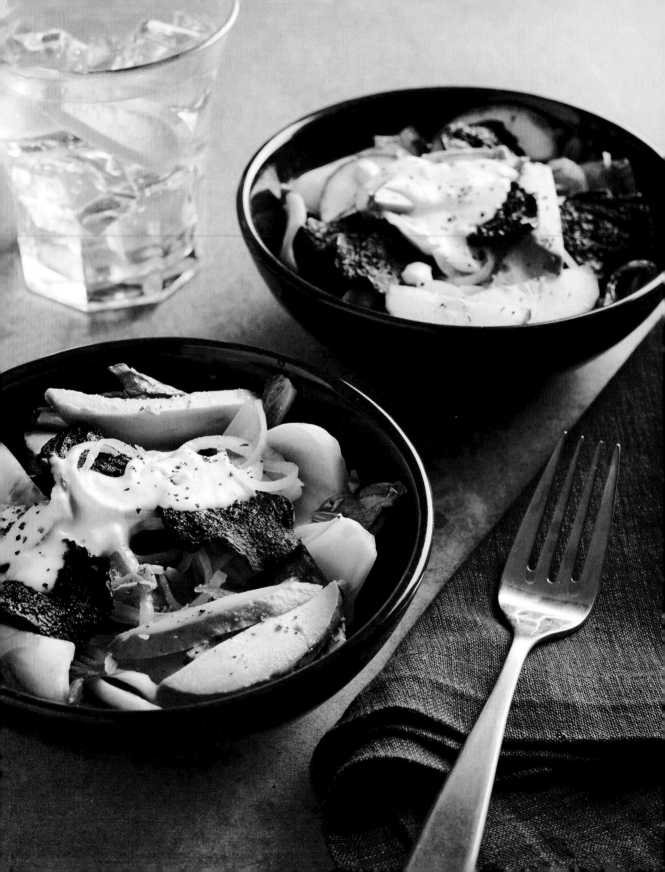

wilted cabbage and beet chip buddha bowls

VEGAN, VEGETARIAN, AIP

START TO FINISH: 40 minutes, plus 2 hours for pickled vegetables

SERVES 2

¼ cup shredded carrots

¼ cup thin slivers sweet onion

¾ teaspoon coarse salt

3 tablespoons fresh lemon juice

2 small beets, trimmed and peeled

4 tablespoons untoasted sesame oil or olive oil

3 cups coarsely shredded savoy cabbage or bok choy

2 garlic cloves, thinly sliced

¼ teaspoon freshly ground black pepper

2 tablespoons coconut cream

½ teaspoon grated fresh ginger or ¼ teaspoon ground ginger

¼ medium English cucumber, halved lengthwise and thinly sliced crosswise (about ¾ cup total)

1 medium avocado, halved, pitted, peeled, and thinly sliced

1 In a small bowl, toss together the carrots, onion, and ⅛ teaspoon salt. Add the juice; toss to coat. Press down to cover as much as possible with the juice. Cover; let sit for 2 hours. Drain, reserving 1 tablespoon of the juice.

2 Preheat the oven to 425°F. Line a baking sheet with parchment paper. Use a mandoline or sharp knife to cut the beets into very thin slices (⅛ inch or thinner). In a medium bowl, toss the beet slices with 1 tablespoon oil and ⅛ teaspoon salt. Arrange in a single layer on the prepared baking sheet.

3 Bake for 14 to 17 minutes, or until crisp and lightly browned. Transfer to a wire rack; cool.

4 In a large skillet, heat 2 tablespoons oil over medium heat. Add the cabbage, garlic, ¼ teaspoon salt, and ⅛ teaspoon pepper. Stir occasionally, for 6 to 8 minutes, or until tender. Remove from the heat.

5 In a small bowl combine the coconut cream, the reserved soaking juice, the ginger, the remaining ⅛ teaspoon salt, and the remaining ⅛ teaspoon pepper. To serve, divide the cabbage between two bowls. Top with the drained carrot mixture and the beet chips, cucumber, and avocado. Dollop with the coconut cream mixture.

Protein: 6 g • **Net Carbs:** 17 g • **Fat:** 43 g

spinach salad

VEGAN, VEGETARIAN

START TO FINISH: 10 minutes

SERVES 2

3 cups fresh baby spinach leaves

1 medium avocado, halved, pitted, peeled, and sliced

¼ cup fresh blueberries

2 tablespoons shelled raw pumpkin seeds (pepitas)

2 teaspoons hemp seeds

1 tablespoon fresh lemon juice

⅛ teaspoon salt

⅛ teaspoon freshly ground black pepper

3 tablespoons extra virgin olive oil

2 teaspoons chopped fresh flat-leaf parsley

1 Divide the spinach between two serving bowls. Top with avocado, blueberries, pumpkin seeds, and hemp seeds.

2 In a small bowl, combine the juice, salt, and pepper. While whisking, drizzle in the olive oil until emulsified. Add the parsley.

3 To serve, drizzle the salads with the dressing.

Protein: 7 g • **Net Carbs:** 5 g • **Fat:** 37 g

roasted eggplant with beet-tahini yogurt and toasted pumpkin seeds

VEGAN, VEGETARIAN

PREP: 15 minutes
ROAST: 15 minutes

SERVES 2

2 tablespoons olive oil, plus extra for greasing

1 small eggplant, cut into four ½- to ¾-inch-thick slices

⅜ teaspoon sea salt

¼ teaspoon freshly ground black pepper

¾ cup plain unsweetened nut milk yogurt

2 ounces packaged cooked beets

1 tablespoon tahini, well stirred

1 teaspoon fresh lemon juice

¼ cup raw unsalted pumpkin seeds, lightly toasted

1 tablespoon minced fresh parsley or cilantro leaves

1 Preheat the oven to 425°F. Brush a parchment paper-lined half-sheet pan generously with oil.

2 Brush both sides of the eggplant slices with 2 tablespoons oil. Sprinkle evenly with ¼ teaspoon salt and ⅛ teaspoon pepper.

3 Place the slices on the sheet pan. Roast for 7 minutes; turn the slices and continue to bake for 7 to 10 minutes or until the eggplant is tender.

4 Meanwhile, in the container of a small food processor, combine the yogurt, beets, tahini, juice, the remaining ⅛ teaspoon salt, and the remaining ⅛ teaspoon pepper. Purée until smooth, about 1 minute.

5 Carefully divide the eggplant slices between two plates. Top with yogurt and sprinkle with pumpkin seeds and parsley.

Protein: 13 g • **Net Carbs:** 11 g • **Fat:** 34 g

---

sheet-pan veggies with nut-free olive-basil pesto

VEGAN, VEGETARIAN, AIP

PREP: 15 minutes
ROAST: 25 minutes

SERVES 2

3 garlic cloves

¼ cup plus 1 teaspoon olive oil

3 cups fresh Brussels sprouts, trimmed and halved

2 cups cremini mushrooms, halved

¾ cup thinly sliced red onion wedges

¼ teaspoon coarse salt

⅜ teaspoon freshly ground black pepper

½ cup pitted green olives

1 cup packed fresh basil leaves

1 to 2 teaspoons finely ground spirulina

1 Preheat the oven to 425°F. Place the garlic on a 4-inch sheet of foil; drizzle with 1 teaspoon oil. Wrap the foil up around the garlic and oil to fully enclose it. Roast the garlic for 20 to 25 minutes, or until the cloves are tender and lightly browned. Cool in the foil pouch on a wire rack.

2 Meanwhile, in a large shallow roasting pan, toss together the Brussels sprouts, mushrooms, onion, 2 tablespoons oil, salt, and ¼ teaspoon pepper. Spread in an even layer. Roast alongside the garlic, uncovered, stirring once or twice, for 25 to 30 minutes, or until the vegetables are tender and golden brown.

3 Transfer the garlic cloves to the container of a blender or food processor. Add the olives. Cover; blend or process until the olives and garlic are finely chopped. Add the basil, spirulina, and the remaining ⅛ teaspoon pepper. Cover and pulse until the basil is finely chopped. Add the remaining 2 tablespoons oil. Cover; blend or process until the pesto is well combined and almost smooth.

4 Divide the roasted vegetables between two serving plates. Drizzle with pesto to serve.

Protein: 9 g • **Net Carbs:** 15 g • **Fat:** 35 g

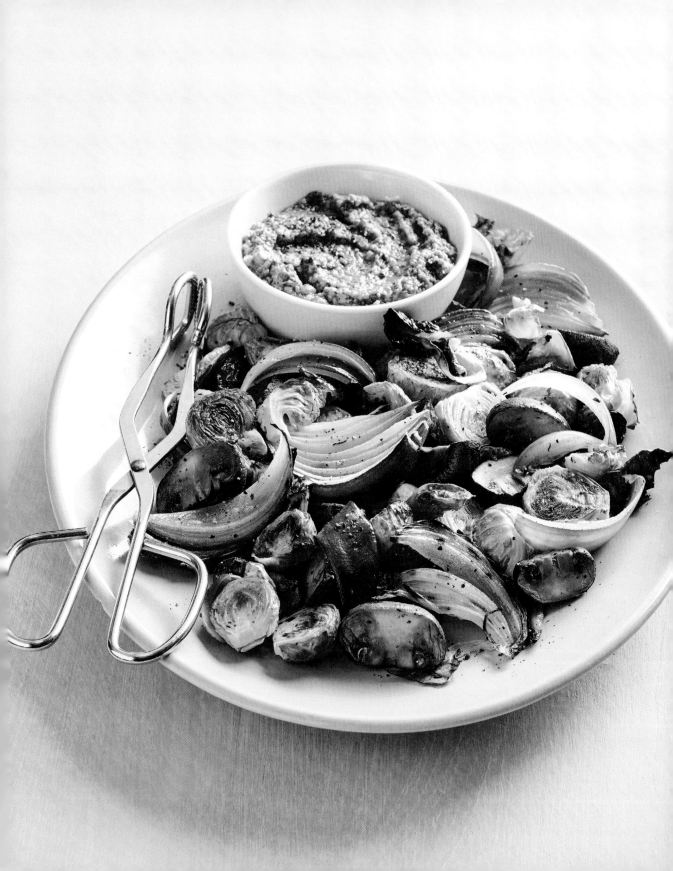

roasted cauliflower tacos

VEGAN, VEGETARIAN, AIP

PREP: 15 minutes
ROAST: 30 minutes

SERVES 2

FOR THE FILLING

4 cups cauliflower florets

¼ cup sliced red onion

2 tablespoons olive oil

¼ teaspoon ground coriander

¼ teaspoon ground cumin

⅛ teaspoon salt

FOR THE SAUCE

1 medium avocado, halved, pitted, peeled, and chopped

¼ cup cilantro leaves and tender stems

2 tablespoons extra virgin olive oil

1 tablespoon fresh lime juice

1 garlic clove, minced

⅛ teaspoon ground cumin

⅛ teaspoon salt

FOR SERVING

6 butterhead or Bibb lettuce leaves

Lime wedges

1 Preheat the oven to 400°F.

2 Place the cauliflower and onion in a medium bowl and drizzle with the oil; mix well to coat. In a small bowl, combine the coriander, cumin, and salt. Sprinkle the spices over the cauliflower and stir to evenly distribute. Spread evenly on a foil-lined large rimmed baking sheet.

3 Roast for 20 minutes; stir. Roast 10 to 15 minutes more, or until the cauliflower is tender and browned.

4 Meanwhile, in the container of a food processor, combine the sauce ingredients. Cover and process until the mixture is smooth. Add water, 1 tablespoon at a time, if the mixture is too thick to blend.

5 Serve the roasted cauliflower mixture in lettuce leaves with avocado sauce and lime wedges.

Protein: 6 g • **Net Carbs:** 12 g • **Fat:** 38 g

---

roasted beets and greens

VEGAN, VEGETARIAN

PREP: 10 minutes
BAKE: 1 hour

SERVES 2

1 red beet

1 golden beet

2 tablespoons coconut oil

¼ pound asparagus, cut into 1-inch pieces

¼ pound escarole, chopped

2 green onions (scallions), sliced

½ teaspoon kosher salt

¼ teaspoon freshly ground black pepper

2 tablespoons chopped walnuts

Vinegar-based hot sauce

1 Preheat the oven to 400°F. Wrap each beet individually in foil. Roast for 1 hour or until easily pierced with a fork.

2 Remove from the oven and allow to cool. Peel the beets, chop off the stem and root, and slice into wedges.

3 Heat a medium skillet over medium-high heat. Add the coconut oil and asparagus and cook for 3 to 5 minutes, until crisp-tender.

4 Add the escarole, green onions, salt, and pepper. Toss to incorporate. Cook for 3 minutes, or until the escarole begins to wilt.

5 Serve the beets on top of the greens. Top with walnuts and hot sauce to taste.

Protein: 5 g • **Net Carbs:** 8 g • **Fat:** 19 g

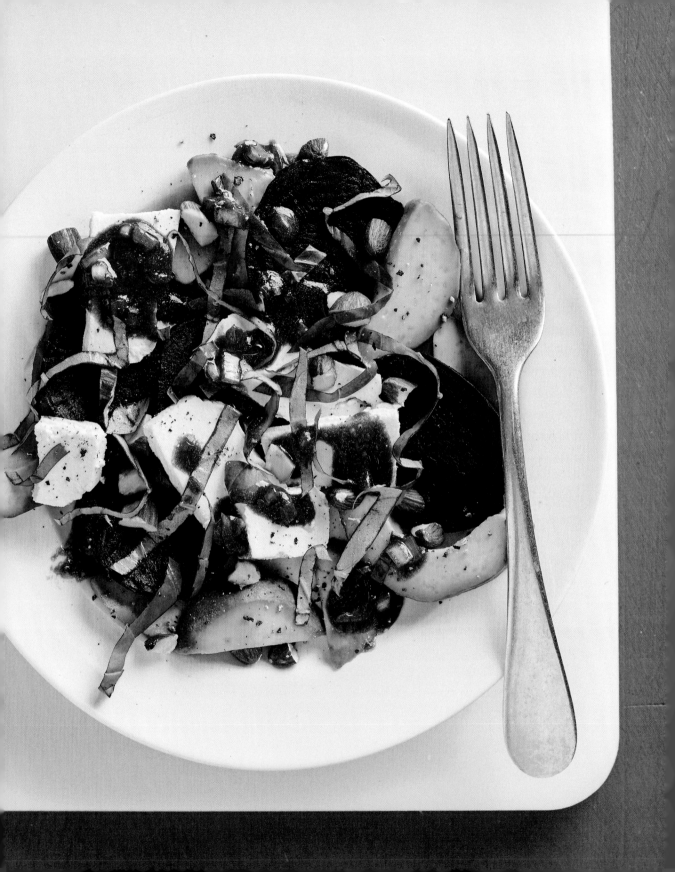

roasted beet–cheese-basil caprese with avocado and toasted almonds

VEGAN, VEGETARIAN

PREP: 10 minutes
ROAST: 1 hour

SERVES 2

1 small beet

2 tablespoons balsamic vinegar

1 tablespoon minced shallots

1 tablespoon extra virgin olive oil

½ teaspoon preservative-free, sugar-free Dijon mustard

¼ teaspoon sea salt

¼ teaspoon freshly ground black pepper

4 ounces soft fresh vegan cheese, sliced

1 small avocado, halved, pitted, peeled, and sliced

¼ cup raw, unsalted almonds, lightly toasted and coarsely chopped

5 fresh basil leaves, thinly sliced

1 Preheat the oven to 400°F. Wrap the beet in foil. Roast until tender when pierced with a fork, about 1 hour. When the beet is cool enough to handle, peel it and cut it into about 8 slices.

2 Meanwhile, in a small bowl, whisk together the vinegar, shallots, oil, mustard, ⅛ teaspoon salt, and ⅛ teaspoon pepper.

3 Arrange the beet, cheese, and avocado slices on two plates and sprinkle with nuts and basil. Sprinkle evenly with the remaining ⅛ teaspoon salt and ⅛ teaspoon pepper, and drizzle evenly with the vinaigrette.

Protein: 12 g • **Net Carbs:** 12 g • **Fat:** 40 g

pesto zoodle bowls

VEGAN, VEGETARIAN

PREP: 15 minutes
COOK: 5 minutes

SERVES 2

FOR THE PESTO

¼ cup olive oil

1½ cups packed fresh baby spinach leaves

½ cup packed fresh basil leaves

¼ cup walnuts

1 garlic clove

⅛ teaspoon salt

FOR THE ZOODLES

2 medium zucchini

1 tablespoon extra virgin olive oil

Dash of freshly ground black pepper

2 ounces soft fresh vegan cheese, crumbled

¼ cup pitted black or green olives, minced

1 In the container of a food processor, combine all of the pesto ingredients. Cover and process until nearly smooth, stopping and scraping the sides as needed.

2 Using a julienne peeler, make long slices along one side of each zucchini until you get down to the seeded core. Rotate the zucchini and continue to peel until you've done all four sides. (If you have a spiralizer, you can use that instead of a julienne peeler.) Discard the core.

3 In a large skillet, heat the oil over medium heat. Add the zoodles and pepper; cook for 3 to 5 minutes, until crisp-tender. Remove from the heat; add the pesto and toss to coat. Divide the mixture between two serving bowls. Top with cheese and olives.

Protein: 9 g • **Net Carbs:** 9 g • **Fat:** 53 g

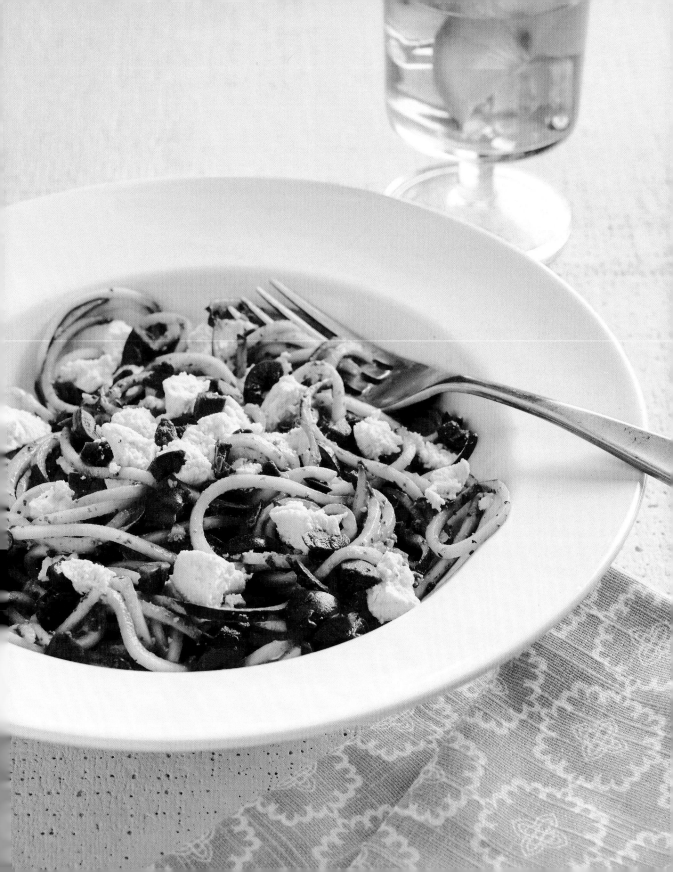

nut-stuffed cremini mushrooms

VEGAN, VEGETARIAN

PREP: 10 minutes
COOK: 20 minutes
COOL: 3 minutes

SERVES 2

½ pound cremini mushrooms

½ cup chopped lightly salted mixed nuts

¼ teaspoon salt

½ teaspoon Chinese five-spice powder

1 tablespoon toasted sesame oil

½ teaspoon sesame seeds

1 tablespoon coconut oil, melted

½ sheet nori, finely chopped

2 tablespoons coarsely chopped parsley leaves

1 Remove the stems of the mushrooms (reserve for another use).

2 In a medium skillet over medium heat, cook the nuts until lightly toasted, about 5 minutes. Add the salt, five-spice powder, sesame oil, and sesame seeds. Cook for 1 minute more. Remove from the heat.

3 Preheat the oven to 375°F. Brush the bottom of a glass baking dish with the coconut oil. Add the mushrooms, top down, and carefully fill with the nut mixture. (The mixture will be hot.) Bake for 15 to 20 minutes, until the mushrooms are soft.

4 Cool for 3 minutes. Sprinkle with nori and parsley before serving.

Protein: 7 g • **Net Carbs:** 8 g • **Fat:** 25 g

individual cauliflower plank pizzas

VEGAN, VEGETARIAN

PREP: 5 minutes
COOK: 30 minutes

SERVES 2 TO 3

1 large head cauliflower

3 tablespoons olive oil

¾ cup chopped fresh cremini or button mushrooms

½ cup chopped red bell pepper

¼ cup chopped red onion

1 garlic clove, minced

⅓ cup pitted green or kalamata olives, chopped

2 teaspoons snipped fresh rosemary or thyme

¼ teaspoon black pepper

½ cup jarred marinara sauce (such as Rao's Homemade Marinara Sauce)

¼ cup soft fresh vegan cheese, crumbled

¼ cup chopped fresh basil leaves

¼ cup vegan ricotta cheese

1 Preheat the oven to 400°F. Line a baking sheet with foil; set aside. Remove the leaves from the cauliflower. Carefully trim the stem end, leaving the core intact so the florets are still attached. Place the cauliflower head core side down. Cut two 1-inch-thick slices from the center of the cauliflower. (Save the rest of the cauliflower for another use.) Place the cauliflower slices on the prepared baking sheet. Brush both sides of the cauliflower slices with 2 tablespoons oil.

2 Roast the cauliflower, uncovered, for 10 minutes. Flip the cauliflower slices. Roast for 10 to 15 minutes more, or until the cauliflower is crisp-tender and starting to brown.

3 Meanwhile, in a medium skillet cook mushrooms, bell pepper, onion, and garlic in remaining 1 tablespoon oil over medium heat, stirring occasionally, for 4 to 5 minutes or until tender and starting to brown. Remove from heat. Stir in olives, rosemary, and black pepper.

4 Spread the marinara sauce evenly on top of the cauliflower slices. Spoon the mushroom mixture evenly over the sauce. Sprinkle with the crumbled cheese. Broil for 3 to 4 minutes, or until the cheese softens.

5 Place pizzas on serving plates. Top with basil and a spoonful of ricotta cheese.

Protein: 8 g • Net Carbs: 13 g • Fat: 31 g

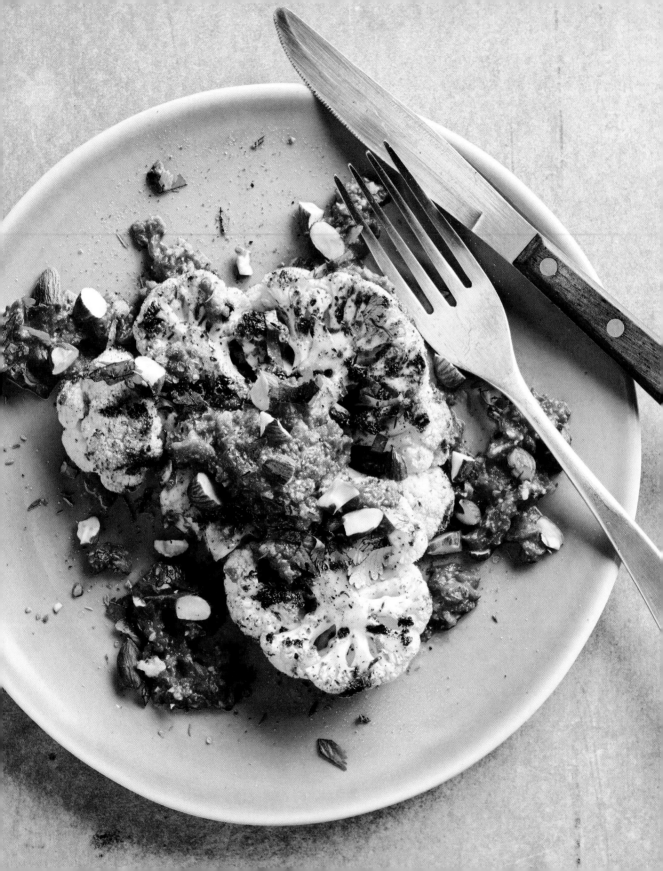

grilled cauliflower steaks with romesco sauce and toasted nuts

VEGAN, VEGETARIAN

PREP: 15 minutes
GRILL: 16 minutes

SERVES 2

One 2¾-pound head cauliflower (for two "steaks")

3 tablespoons olive oil

2 tablespoons sherry vinegar

¼ teaspoon ras el hanout seasoning

½ teaspoon sea salt

¼ cup raw unsalted almonds, lightly toasted and chopped

¼ cup roasted red bell peppers, drained

1 teaspoon minced fresh garlic

⅛ teaspoon freshly ground black pepper

2 tablespoons finely chopped fresh parsley leaves

1 Preheat the grill to medium-high heat (350°F to 400°F). Hold the cauliflower head stalk side down on a cutting board. Cut the cauliflower into 1½-inch-thick slabs all the way across, yielding two large "steaks" from the middle of the head, and florets from the edges. Trim and discard the green parts from the steaks and the bottom inch of the stalk. (Reserve the florets for another use.) Pat both sides of the steaks dry.

2 Whisk 2 tablespoons oil, 1 tablespoon vinegar, the ras el hanout seasoning, and ¼ teaspoon salt until thoroughly combined.

3 Brush the cauliflower steaks with approximately half of the olive oil mixture.

4 Grill the steaks, covered, on well-oiled grill grates for 8 minutes, until slightly charred. Turn and brush with the remaining oil mixture. Cover and continue to grill for 8 to 10 minutes, or until the cauliflower is tender but not mushy. Remove from the grill; cover with foil and keep warm.

recipe continues

5 Meanwhile, add the remaining 1 tablespoon oil, the remaining 1 tablespoon vinegar, 2 tablespoons almonds, bell peppers, garlic, the remaining ¼ teaspoon salt, and the black pepper to the container of a small food processor and purée until almost smooth, about 1 minute. Finely chop the remaining 2 tablespoons almonds and set aside.

6 Divide the sauce between the steaks. Sprinkle with the remaining 2 tablespoons chopped almonds and the parsley.

Protein: 8 g • **Net Carbs:** 9 g • **Fat:** 30 g

---

butter cauliflower

VEGETARIAN

PREP: 5 minutes
SOAK: Overnight
COOK: 25 minutes

SERVES 4

½ cup raw whole cashews

1 can (14.5 ounces) diced tomatoes, undrained

⅓ cup ghee

½ cup chopped white onion

2 garlic cloves, minced

2 teaspoons minced fresh ginger

1 to 2 teaspoons garam masala

¼ teaspoon salt

⅛ teaspoon cayenne pepper

6 cups small cauliflower florets

⅔ cup full-fat coconut milk

2 tablespoons chopped fresh cilantro

½ cup toasted cashews

1 Place the raw whole cashews in a small bowl and cover with cold water. Refrigerate overnight. Drain and rinse the cashews; place in the container of a blender with the tomatoes. Cover and blend until smooth, scraping the sides as needed; set aside.

2 In a large nonstick skillet, heat the ghee over medium heat. Add the onion and cook, stirring occasionally, for 2 to 3 minutes, until softened. Add the garlic, ginger, garam masala, salt, and cayenne; cook and stir for 1 minute, until fragrant. Stir in the cauliflower and the cashew-tomato mixture. Bring to a boil. Reduce the heat to low and simmer, covered, for 10 to 12 minutes or until the cauliflower is tender, stirring occasionally. Stir in the coconut milk; heat through. Remove from the heat; stir in the cilantro. Sprinkle with the toasted cashews.

Protein: 10 g • **Net Carbs:** 22 g • **Fat:** 40 g

coconut mushroom simmer

VEGAN, VEGETARIAN

PREP: 5 minutes
COOK: 6 minutes

SERVES 3

2 tablespoons coarsely chopped fresh lemongrass*

2 Thai or Fresno chilies, stemmed and coarsely chopped (leave seeds in for more heat)

3 garlic cloves, peeled

2 tablespoons coarsely chopped fresh cilantro leaves

1 teaspoon freshly ground black pepper

1 teaspoon kosher salt

2 tablespoons coconut oil

¼ cup raw cashews

1 zucchini, cubed (2 cups)

2 cups full-fat coconut milk

1 cup shiitake mushrooms, stemmed and sliced

1 cup oyster mushrooms, halved

½ cup enoki mushrooms, for topping

Lemon wedges

1 Combine the lemongrass, chilies, garlic, cilantro, pepper, and salt in a mortar and pestle or spice grinder; crush or pulse until it forms a coarsely textured paste.

2 Heat the coconut oil in a medium skillet over medium heat. Add the cashews and zucchini and cook, stirring occasionally, for 2 minutes.

3 Stir in the lemongrass paste and cook for 1 minute, stirring constantly.

4 Add the coconut milk and the shiitake and oyster mushrooms; simmer for 3 minutes.

5 Serve topped with the enoki mushrooms and a squeeze of lemon.

Protein: 8 g • **Net Carbs:** 16 g • **Fat:** 36 g

---

*NOTE: To prepare lemongrass for cooking, trim off the bottom of the stalk and the woody leaves—about two-thirds of the stalk's length. Peel away and discard any tough outer layers. Coarsely chop the core.

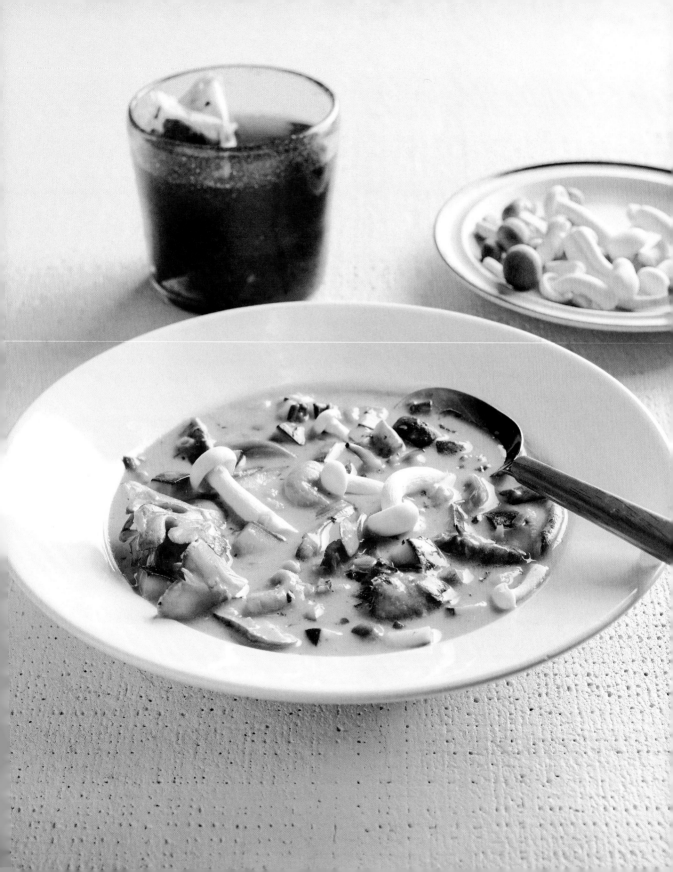

cauliflower hummus wraps

VEGAN, VEGETARIAN

PREP: 8 minutes
COOL: 15 minutes
COOK: 20 minutes

SERVES 2

FOR THE HUMMUS

4 cups cauliflower florets

2 garlic cloves

4 tablespoons olive oil

¼ teaspoon salt

Dash of cayenne pepper

2 tablespoons tahini, well stirred

1 tablespoon fresh lemon juice

FOR SERVING

6 large butterhead or Bibb lettuce leaves

¼ cup seeded and chopped tomato

¼ cup chopped cucumber

2 tablespoons pitted black olives, coarsely chopped

2 tablespoons tahini, well stirred

1 Preheat the oven to 400°F.

2 Place the cauliflower and garlic in a medium bowl and drizzle with 2 tablespoons oil; mix well to coat. Add the salt and cayenne; mix well. Spread evenly on a large rimmed baking sheet.

3 Roast for 10 minutes; stir. Roast 10 to 15 minutes more, or until the cauliflower is tender and beginning to brown. Cool for 15 minutes.

4 In the container of a food processor, combine the roasted cauliflower mixture, the remaining 2 tablespoons oil, and the tahini and juice. Cover and process until smooth, stopping and scraping the sides as needed. If the mixture is too thick, add water, 1 tablespoon at a time, until the desired consistency is reached.

5 Serve the cauliflower hummus in lettuce leaves topped with tomato, cucumber, and olives. Drizzle with tahini.

Protein: 10 g • **Net Carbs:** 14 g • **Fat:** 45 g

breakfast

Here are simple and yummy breakfasts to start your day off with sustainable energy to get you through the morning and beyond. When you are in a healthy fat-adapted state, however, breakfast is far from the most important meal. Whenever you feel like it, skip breakfast and do an intermittent fast (autophagy, anyone?). Ketotarianism offers you freedom to make the healthiest food choices for your body. And of course, you can always use these breakfast recipes for lunch or dinner too (you're such a rebel).

asparagus scramble

VEGETARIAN

START TO FINISH: 15 minutes

SERVES 2

2 tablespoons olive oil

½ cup 1-inch pieces fresh asparagus

2 tablespoons chopped red bell pepper

4 large eggs

⅛ teaspoon salt

⅛ teaspoon freshly ground black pepper

¼ cup nut-based soft fresh vegan cheese

2 teaspoons chopped fresh chives

1 In a large nonstick skillet, heat the oil over medium heat. Add the asparagus and bell pepper; cook for 3 to 4 minutes, until the vegetables are tender.

2 Meanwhile, in a medium bowl, whisk together the eggs, salt, black pepper, and 2 tablespoons water. Pour the egg mixture into the skillet. Cook over medium heat, without stirring, until the mixture begins to set on the bottom and around the edges. With a spatula, lift and fold the partially cooked egg mixture so the uncooked portion flows underneath. Continue cooking for 1 to 2 minutes, until the egg mixture is cooked through.

3 Divide the scrambled eggs between two plates. Top with spoonfuls of cheese and sprinkle with chives.

Protein: 15 g • **Net Carbs:** 3 g • **Fat:** 27 g

berry-cream parfaits with toasted coconut topping

VEGAN, VEGETARIAN

PREP: 20 minutes
BAKE: 5 minutes

SERVES 2

½ cup shredded unsweetened coconut

2 tablespoons coconut oil, melted

⅛ teaspoon ground cinnamon

⅛ teaspoon ground cardamom

⅛ teaspoon sea salt

1 cup mixed blueberries and raspberries

¾ cup plain unsweetened almond-milk or coconut-milk yogurt (5.3-ounce carton)

¾ cup unsweetened coconut cream, well stirred (5.4-ounce can)

1 Preheat the oven to 300°F. Line a half-sheet pan with parchment paper. In a medium bowl, toss the coconut with the oil, cinnamon, cardamom, and salt. Bake, stirring halfway through, for 5 to 6 minutes, until light golden in spots and aromatic. Let cool to room temperature, about 15 minutes.

2 In each of two parfait or lowball glasses, layer half each of the berries, yogurt, coconut cream, and toasted coconut mixture. Repeat the layers, ending with the coconut.

NOTE: For an AIP-compliant recipe, use coconut-milk yogurt.

Protein: 5 g • **Net Carbs:** 17 g • **Fat:** 55 g

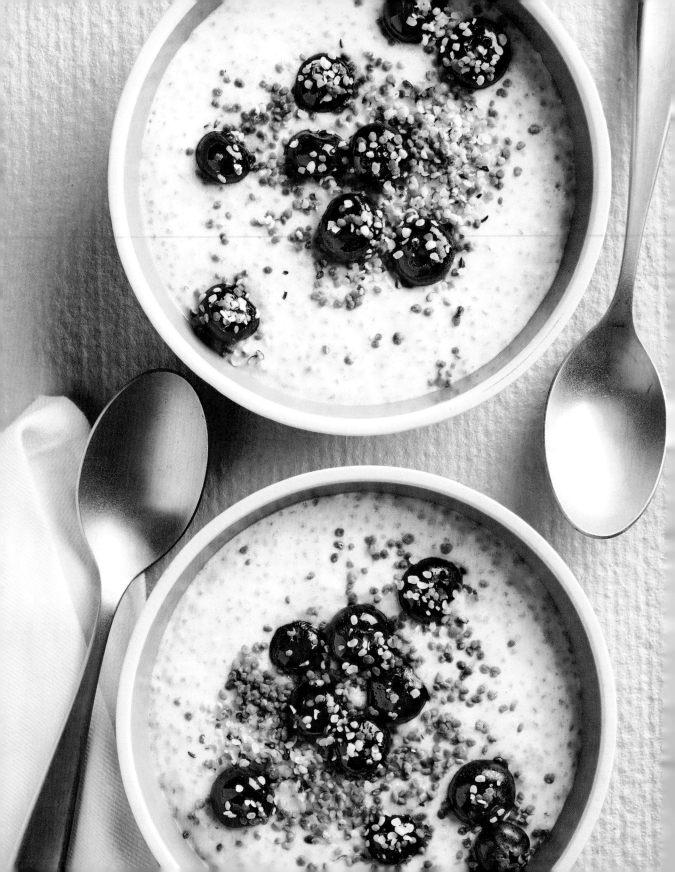

chia pudding breakfast bowls

VEGETARIAN

PREP: 5 minutes
CHILL: 20 minutes

SERVES 2

¼ cup unsweetened almond milk*

¾ cup full-fat coconut milk

¼ teaspoon vanilla extract

4 drops liquid stevia

2 tablespoons chia seeds

1 tablespoon hemp protein powder

½ cup fresh blueberries

2 teaspoons bee pollen

2 tablespoons hemp seeds

1 In a medium bowl, whisk together the almond milk, coconut milk, vanilla, and stevia. Add the chia seeds and hemp protein powder; whisk to combine. Refrigerate for 20 minutes, whisking occasionally to distribute the chia seeds, until the chia seeds have absorbed the liquid and the mixture has thickened.

2 Divide the pudding between two bowls. Top with the blueberries, bee pollen, and hemp seeds.

Protein: 11 g • Net Carbs: 9 g • Fat: 23 g

*TIP: To make your own almond milk, combine 1½ cups water and 1½ cups raw unsalted almonds in a medium bowl. Cover and let stand 12 to 48 hours (the longer it stands, the richer and creamier the milk will be). Drain the nuts, discarding the liquids. Rinse and drain. In the container of a blender, combine the soaked almonds, 3 cups water, and ¼ teaspoon salt. Cover and blend on high for 2 minutes. Line a colander with two layers of cheesecloth and set over a large bowl. Strain the almond mixture through the colander, bringing up the corners of the cheesecloth and gently squeezing to release the liquid. Discard the solids. If desired, stir in 1 teaspoon vanilla. Store in the refrigerator for up to 1 week. Stir before using.

egg-o-cado

VEGAQUARIAN

PREP: 5 minutes
BAKE: 15 minutes

SERVES 2

1 large avocado, halved
and pitted

Olive oil

2 medium eggs

2 ounces lox salmon, coarsely
chopped

1½ teaspoons chopped fresh
chives

¼ teaspoon kosher salt

½ teaspoon coarsely ground
black pepper

½ lemon

Crushed red pepper, to garnish

1 Preheat the oven to 400°F.

2 Gently remove 1 tablespoon avocado flesh from
each half, reserving for other use.

3 Lightly oil a sheet pan with olive oil. Arrange
each avocado half on the pan and press it so
it lies flat. Carefully crack one egg into each
avocado half.

4 Bake for 15 to 20 minutes, or until the whites
are set and the yolk has reached the desired
consistency.

5 Top with lox, chives, salt, and pepper. Squeeze
lemon juice to taste over the eggs and garnish
with the crushed red pepper.

Protein: 13 g • **Net Carbs:** 2 g • **Fat:** 23 g

NOTE: To make this vegetarian, leave off the lox.

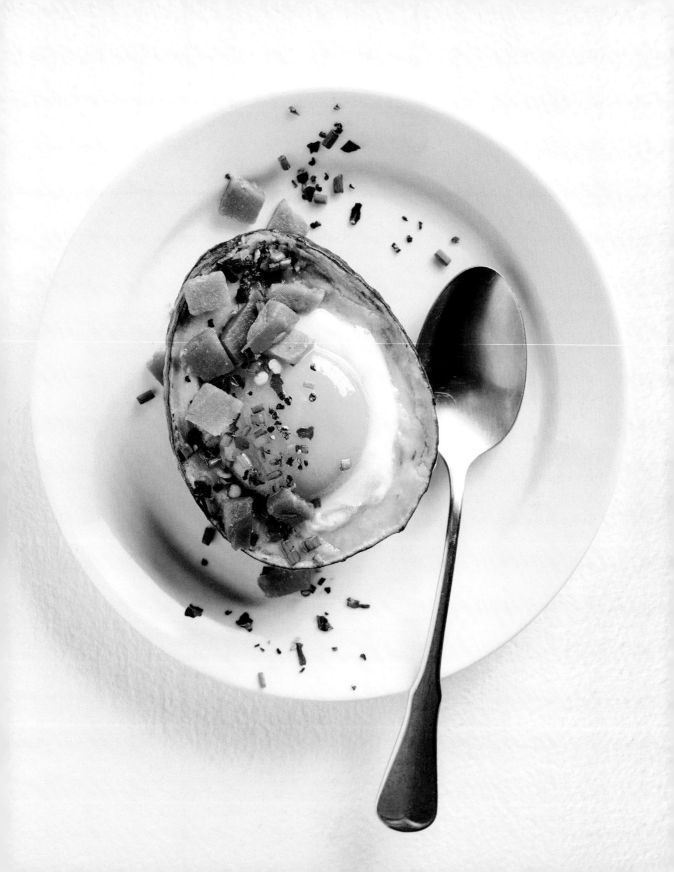

lox and egg scramble with dilled almond-milk yogurt

VEGAQUARIAN

START TO FINISH: 15 minutes

SERVES 2

¼ cup plain unsweetened almond-milk yogurt

2 teaspoons finely chopped fresh dill

⅛ teaspoon sea salt

⅛ teaspoon freshly ground black pepper

3 large eggs

6 ounces smoked salmon, diced

1 tablespoon ghee

1 In a small bowl, stir together the yogurt, dill, salt, and half of the pepper.

2 In a medium bowl, whisk the eggs. Stir in the salmon and the remaining pepper until well-blended.

2 In a small nonstick skillet, melt the ghee over medium heat. Add the egg mixture and reduce the heat to medium-low. Cook, stirring frequently with a wooden spoon to form small curds, for 4 to 5 minutes, until mostly cooked through. Turn off the heat and let the eggs continue cooking in the pan for 1 minute more.

4 Divide the eggs between two plates and top each portion with half of the yogurt.

Protein: 26 g • **Net Carbs:** 1 g • **Fat:** 20 g

quick egg-chard scramble

VEGETARIAN

START TO FINISH: 15 minutes

SERVES 2

2 fresh rainbow chard or regular chard leaves

2 tablespoons refined coconut oil or avocado oil

¼ cup slivered red onion

3 large eggs

¼ teaspoon coarse salt

¼ teaspoon ground mustard

⅛ to ¼ teaspoon freshly ground black pepper

2 tablespoons snipped fresh parsley or basil leaves or 1 tablespoon snipped fresh chives

1 Trim the stems from the chard leaves. Thinly slice the stems. Coarsely chop the leaves; set the leaves aside. In a medium skillet, heat 1 tablespoon oil over medium heat and add the sliced chard stems and onion. Cook for 3 to 5 minutes, or until the vegetables are tender, stirring occasionally. Add the chard leaves. Cook and stir for 1 to 2 minutes more, or just until the chard leaves are wilted and tender. Push the vegetables to the edge of the skillet.

2 Meanwhile, in a medium bowl, beat the eggs, salt, mustard, and pepper with a whisk until well combined. Add the remaining 1 tablespoon oil to the center of the skillet. Add the egg mixture to the center of the skillet. Cook over medium-low heat, without stirring, until the mixture begins to set on the bottom and around the edges.

3 Using a spatula or large spoon, lift and fold the partially cooked egg mixture so the uncooked portion flows underneath. Continue cooking for 2 to 3 minutes, or until the egg mixture is cooked through but is still glossy and moist. Stir the chard mixture into the scrambled eggs. Remove from the heat. Sprinkle with parsley.

Protein: 11 g • **Net Carbs:** 3 g • **Fat:** 21 g

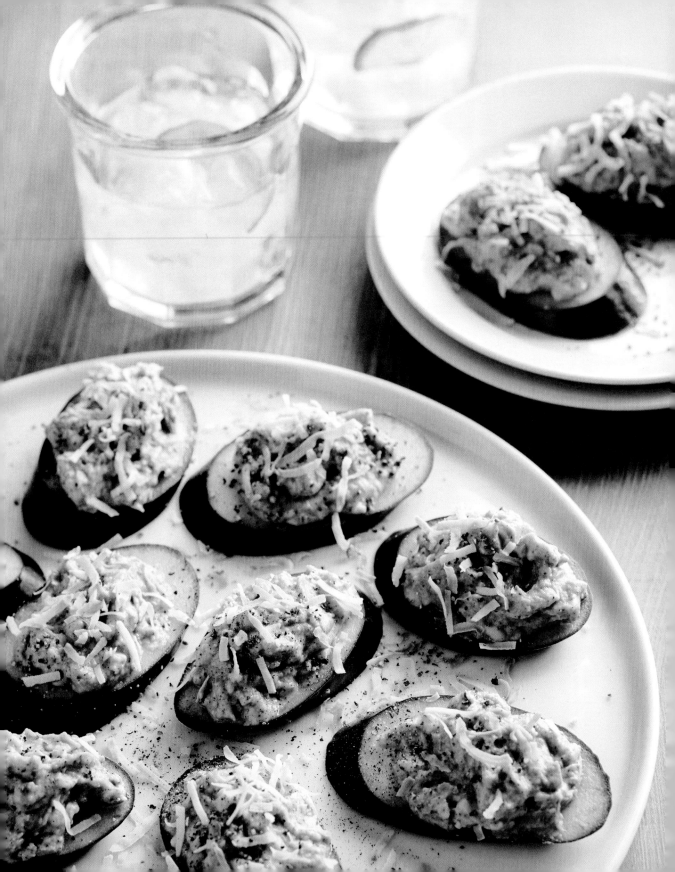

cucumber "toast" bites with avocado and coconut

VEGAN, VEGETARIAN

START TO FINISH: 20 minutes

SERVES 2

1 large avocado, halved, pitted, and peeled

3 tablespoons canned coconut milk

2 teaspoons finely ground spirulina

⅛ teaspoon salt

¼ teaspoon crushed red pepper

1 tablespoon hemp protein powder

Sixteen ¼-inch-thick cucumber slices

3 tablespoons unsweetened shredded coconut, toasted

Freshly ground black pepper

In a medium bowl combine the avocado, coconut milk, spirulina, salt, crushed red pepper, and hemp protein powder. Mash with a potato masher or fork until well combined and smooth. Spoon the avocado mixture evenly atop the cucumber slices. Sprinkle with the coconut and black pepper.

Protein: 7 g • Net Carbs: 8 g • Fat: 18 g

roasted beet with avocado, grapefruit, and pickled red onion

VEGAN, VEGETARIAN, AIP

PREP: 25 minutes

ROAST: 1 hour

SERVES 2

1 medium golden beet

3 tablespoons cider vinegar

3 tablespoons avocado oil

⅛ teaspoon chili powder

⅛ teaspoon sea salt, plus additional for seasoning

Dash of ground cloves

Dash of ground mustard

Dash of freshly ground black pepper

½ small red onion, thinly sliced

1 large avocado, halved, pitted, peeled, and cut into 8 slices

½ medium ruby red grapefruit, cut into sections

1 Preheat the oven to 400°F. Wrap the beet tightly in foil and roast until tender, about 1 hour. When the beet is cool enough to handle, peel it and cut it into eight slices. (You can roast the beet a day ahead and refrigerated until ready to assemble the dish.)

2 In a medium bowl, whisk 2 tablespoons vinegar with the oil, chili powder, and ⅛ teaspoon salt. Add the beet slices, toss well, and let marinate at room temperature for about 20 minutes.

3 Meanwhile, in a small bowl, whisk together the remaining 1 tablespoon vinegar and a dash each of salt, cloves, mustard, and pepper. Add the onion and let it marinate at room temperature for 20 minutes.

4 When ready to assemble, drain the beet and onion (discard the marinades). On each of two plates, arrange the beet slices, pickled onion, avocado, and grapefruit. Sprinkle the avocado and grapefruit evenly with salt to taste.

Protein: 3 g • Net Carbs: 11 g • Fat: 32 g

eggs for dinner

Who says eggs are only for breakfast? Organic fresh eggs are a simple, nutrient-dense food that is incredibly (and edibly) versatile. Why limit this delicious omega-fat-and-vitamin-rich food to the mornings? Enjoy these creative, fun options any time of the day.

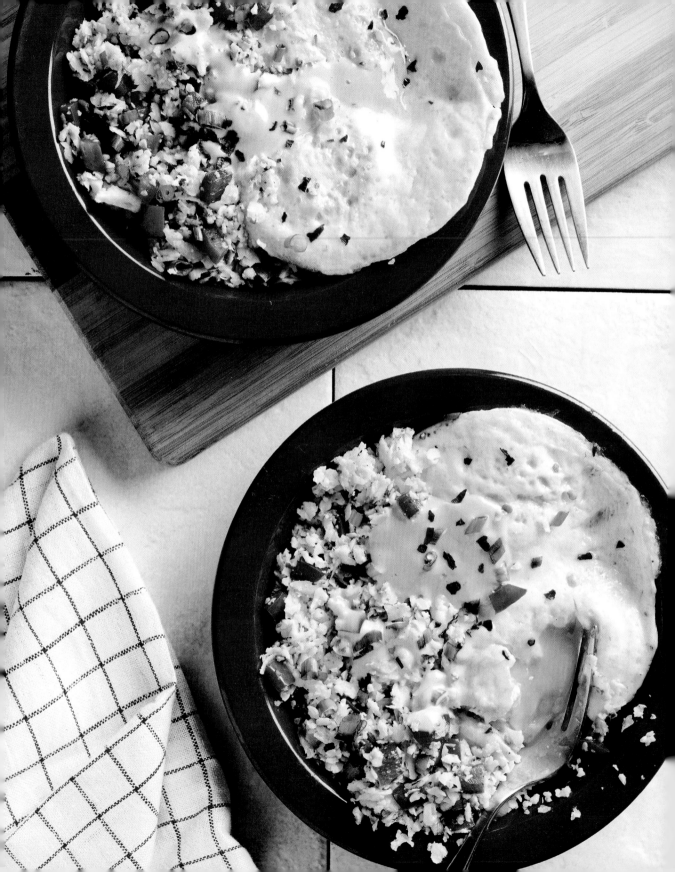

cauliflower fried rice bowls

VEGETARIAN

PREP: 5 minutes
COOK: 12 minutes

SERVES 2

3 tablespoons olive oil

One 16-ounce bag riced fresh cauliflower (4 cups)

½ cup chopped red bell pepper

2 green onions (scallions), sliced, white and green parts separated

1 garlic clove, minced

⅛ teaspoon salt

Dash of red pepper flakes

4 teaspoons coconut aminos

4 large eggs

3 tablespoons avocado-oil mayonnaise

1 In a large skillet, heat 2 tablespoons oil over medium-high heat. Add the cauliflower, bell pepper, green onion whites, garlic, salt, and red pepper flakes. Cook for 6 to 8 minutes, or until the vegetables are tender, stirring often. Stir in 3 teaspoons coconut aminos. Divide the cauliflower mixture between two serving bowls.

2 In the same skillet, heat the remaining 1 tablespoon oil over medium heat. Break the eggs into the skillet. Reduce the heat to low. Cover the eggs and cook for 3 to 4 minutes, or until the whites are completely set and the yolks start to thicken. Turn the eggs and cook for 30 seconds more for over-easy fried eggs.

3 Meanwhile, in a small bowl, stir together the mayonnaise and the remaining 1 teaspoon coconut aminos.

4 Serve the fried eggs over the cauliflower mixture. Top with the mayonnaise mixture and the green onion greens.

Protein: 19g • **Net Carbs:** 10 g • **Fat:** 49 g

chinese fried
cabbage-and-egg-stuffed peppers

VEGETARIAN

PREP: 5 minutes
COOK: 20 minutes

SERVES 2

2 medium red bell peppers, halved from top to bottom (leave stem on), seeded

2 cups coarsely shredded green cabbage

1 small shallot, cut into thin slivers

1 carrot, finely chopped

2 tablespoons toasted sesame oil

1 tablespoon liquid aminos

2 teaspoons finely chopped fresh ginger

⅛ to ¼ teaspoon red pepper flakes

1 tablespoon untoasted sesame oil or refined coconut oil

3 large eggs, lightly beaten

2 teaspoons toasted sesame seeds, plus more as garnish (optional)

1 Place a steamer basket in a 4-to-6-quart saucepan or pot. Add enough water to almost touch the bottom of the basket. Bring to a boil. Add bell peppers to basket. Cover; steam for 6 to 8 minutes, or until just tender. Remove peppers. Invert on paper towels to drain.

2 Meanwhile, in a large skillet, cook the cabbage, shallot, and carrot in the toasted sesame oil for 6 to 8 minutes, or until the cabbage is wilted and the carrot is just tender, stirring frequently. Stir in the liquid aminos, ginger, and red pepper flakes. Reduce the heat to medium-low. Push the cabbage mixture to the edges of the skillet.

3 Add the untoasted sesame oil to the center of the skillet. Add the beaten eggs to the center of the skillet. Cook over medium-low heat, without stirring, until the mixture begins to set. With a spatula or large spoon, lift and fold the partially cooked egg mixture so that the uncooked portion flows underneath. Continue cooking for 3 to 4 minutes, or until the egg is cooked through but still glossy and moist. Sprinkle with sesame seeds, if using. Stir to combine the eggs with the cabbage mixture.

4 To serve, place bell pepper halves on each serving plate. Evenly spoon in the cabbage mixture. Sprinkle with sesame seeds, if desired.

Protein: 14 g • **Net Carbs:** 12 g • **Fat:** 29 g

omelet with sautéed mushrooms, chard, and nut cheese

VEGETARIAN

PREP: 10 minutes
COOK: 15 minutes

SERVES 2

3 tablespoons ghee

2 tablespoons minced red onion

2 garlic cloves, minced

4 ounces shiitake mushrooms, stems removed (and discarded) and caps thinly sliced

½ teaspoon minced fresh thyme leaves

¼ teaspoon sea salt

¼ teaspoon freshly ground black pepper

1 cup Swiss chard leaves (ideally from red chard), very thinly sliced

2 teaspoons cider vinegar

5 large eggs

2 tablespoons plain unsweetened almond or cashew milk

4 ounces soft fresh vegan cheese, sliced or crumbled

1 In a medium skillet, heat 1½ tablespoons ghee over medium-high heat. Once hot, add the onion and garlic and sauté until the onion is translucent, about 2 minutes. Add the mushrooms, thyme, ⅛ teaspoon salt, and ⅛ teaspoon pepper. Sauté until the mushrooms are golden brown and tender and the liquid has evaporated, about 4 minutes. Add the chard and sauté until completely wilted, about 1 minute. Add the vinegar and simmer for 1 minute. Set aside.

2 Meanwhile, in a medium bowl, whisk together the eggs, milk, the remaining ⅛ teaspoon salt, and the remaining ⅛ teaspoon pepper.

3 Heat the remaining 1½ tablespoons ghee in a 12-inch nonstick skillet over medium-high heat. Add the egg mixture and cook, undisturbed, for about 2 minutes. Then, once the eggs just begin to set on the sides, use a wooden spoon to gently scrape any liquid eggs from the sides to the center of the pan.

4 Once the center of the eggs begins to set, top with the vegetable mixture and cheese. Cook for another 2 minutes. Cover with a lid and remove from the heat. Let stand for 2 minutes to soften the cheese. Fold in half and slide onto a cutting board. Cut into two pieces and serve immediately.

Protein: 24 g • **Net Carbs:** 9 g • **Fat:** 49 g

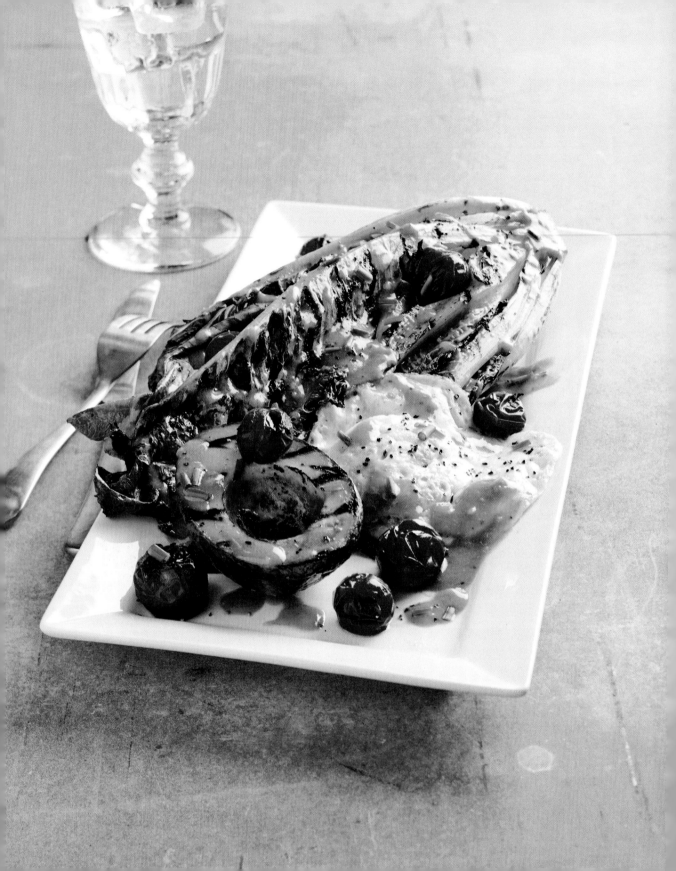

grilled romaine and avocado caesar salad with eggs

VEGAQUARIAN

PREP: 15 minutes
COOK: 10 minutes

SERVES 2

2 teaspoons finely chopped anchovies

1 small garlic clove, minced

⅜ teaspoon coarse salt

1 tablespoon fresh lemon juice

1 teaspoon Dijon mustard

5 tablespoons olive oil

1 romaine heart, halved lengthwise

1 large avocado, halved and pitted

1½ cups cherry tomatoes (1 pint)

2 teaspoons ghee

2 large eggs

⅛ teaspoon coarse salt

⅛ teaspoon freshly ground black pepper, plus more to taste

Chopped fresh chives

1 Prepare two 10-to-12-inch skewers; if using bamboo skewers, soak them in water for at least 30 minutes.

2 On a cutting board, use the side of a chef's knife to mash the anchovies, garlic, and ¼ teaspoon salt into a paste. Transfer to a medium bowl. Add the juice and mustard. Whisk until well combined. While whisking, very slowly add 3 tablespoons oil in a thin stream until the dressing is thickened and well combined. Set the dressing aside.

3 Brush the cut sides of the romaine and avocado with 1 tablespoon oil. Toss the tomatoes with the remaining 1 tablespoon olive oil. Thread the tomatoes onto the skewers. For a charcoal grill, place the romaine and avocado, cut sides down, on the rack directly over medium coals. Place the skewers on the rack directly over medium coals. Grill the romaine and avocado for 2 to 3 minutes, or until lightly charred. Grill the skewers for 4 to 6 minutes, or until lightly charred, turning once halfway through grilling. (For a gas grill, preheat the grill. Reduce the heat to medium. Place the romaine, avocado, and skewers on the grill rack over the heat as directed. Cover and grill as directed.)

recipe continues

4 Meanwhile, in a medium skillet, heat the ghee over medium heat. Break the eggs into the skillet, leaving space between the eggs. Sprinkle with the remaining ⅛ teaspoon salt and ⅛ teaspoon pepper. Reduce the heat to low. Cook the eggs for 3 to 4 minutes, or until the whites are completely set and the yolks start to thicken. Flip the eggs. Cook for 30 seconds more, or until the yolks are cooked to the desired doneness.

5 Divide the romaine, avocado, and tomatoes between two serving plates. Top with a fried egg. Drizzle with the dressing. Sprinkle with pepper and chives.

Protein: 11 g • **Net Carbs:** 7 g • **Fat:** 55 g

---

greens frittata

VEGETARIAN

PREP: 10 minutes
COOK: 10 minutes

SERVES 4

4 ounces purple or curly-leaf green kale leaves, stems removed, coarsely torn

4 ounces fresh baby spinach leaves

1 head baby bok choy, coarsely chopped

6 large eggs, beaten

¼ cup coconut cream

2 garlic cloves, crushed

1 celery stick, cut into small dice (¼ cup)

1 shallot, cut into small dice

2 Fresno chilies or 1 jalapeño chili, seeds and ribs removed, minced

1 teaspoon chopped fresh oregano leaves or ¼ teaspoon dried oregano leaves

¼ teaspoon sea salt

3 tablespoons olive oil

½ cup chopped pecans

¼ cup soft fresh vegan cheese, crumbled

1 teaspoon Spanish paprika

1 Preheat the broiler to high and position the upper rack 6 inches below the broiler.

2 Heat a large, heavy skillet over medium heat. Add the kale, spinach, bok choy, and ¼ cup water. Cook until wilted, about 3 minutes. Drain and pat dry with paper towels.

3 Whisk together the eggs, coconut cream, garlic, celery, shallot, chilies, oregano, and salt in a large bowl. Stir in the greens.

4 Heat a large, heavy, oven-safe skillet over medium-high heat. Add the oil. Tilt the pan to ensure that the entire surface is oiled.

5 Gently pour in the egg mixture. Top with the pecans and cheese. Without stirring, cook for 6 minutes, until the sides begin to set.

6 Finish under the broiler for about 3 minutes, or until the eggs are firm.

7 Sprinkle with paprika and let rest for 3 minutes before slicing and serving.

Protein: 15 g • **Net Carbs:** 8 g • **Fat:** 35 g

spicy frittata pizza
with spinach and olives

VEGETARIAN

PREP: 15 minutes
COOK: 13 minutes

SERVES 2

5 large eggs

2 tablespoons plain unsweetened almond milk

¼ teaspoon sea salt

⅛ teaspoon freshly ground black pepper

1 tablespoon olive oil

2 teaspoon minced garlic

⅛ teaspoon red pepper flakes

8 ounces fresh baby spinach leaves, washed well and spun dry

4 ounces soft fresh vegan cheese, sliced or crumbled

8 pitted kalamata or niçoise olives, halved

6 fresh basil leaves, finely chopped

1 Preheat the oven to 375°F.

2 In a medium bowl, whisk together the eggs, milk, ⅛ teaspoon salt, and ⅛ teaspoon black pepper.

3 Heat the oil in a medium oven-safe nonstick skillet over medium-high heat. When hot, add the garlic and red pepper flakes. Cook for 2 minutes (do not let it brown). Add the spinach, the remaining ⅛ teaspoon salt, and the remaining ⅛ teaspoon black pepper. Cook, stirring frequently, until the spinach is wilted, about 2 minutes.

4 Immediately pour the eggs into the pan and reduce the heat to medium. Sprinkle the cheese and olives evenly over the top. Cook until the edges of the eggs are just set, about 3 minutes.

5 Carefully transfer the pan to the oven and bake until the eggs are cooked through, 5 to 8 minutes. Sprinkle with basil and serve.

Protein: 25 g • **Net Carbs:** 8 g • **Fat:** 37 g

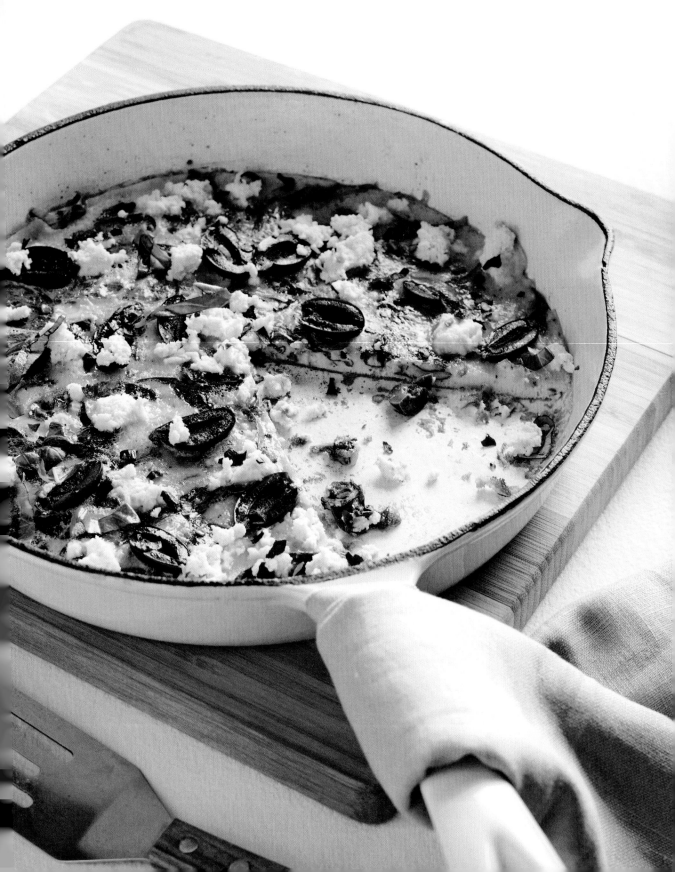

italian egg-stuffed portobello mushrooms

VEGETARIAN

PREP: 20 minutes
COOK: 40 minutes

SERVES 2

1 cup cherry tomatoes

1 cup chopped, peeled eggplant

½ cup chopped red bell pepper

⅓ cup chopped red onion

1 garlic clove, chopped

¼ teaspoon coarse salt, plus more to taste

⅛ teaspoon freshly ground black pepper, plus more to taste

4 tablespoons olive oil

2 large portobello mushrooms (5 to 6 ounces each)

2 medium eggs

3 tablespoons pitted kalamata olives, chopped

1 tablespoon snipped fresh oregano

2 teaspoons balsamic vinegar

Chopped fresh basil leaves

1 Preheat the oven to 425°F. In a 3-quart rectangular baking dish, combine the tomatoes, eggplant, bell pepper, onion, garlic, ¼ teaspoon salt, and ⅛ teaspoon pepper. Drizzle with 2 tablespoons oil; toss to coat. Roast uncovered, stirring once or twice, for 25 to 30 minutes, or until the vegetables are tender and lightly charred.

2 Meanwhile, line a small baking sheet with parchment paper or foil. Remove the stems from the mushrooms. Using a spoon, gently scrape out the gills; discard. Scoop out the center of each mushroom (approximately 2 tablespoons) to make a small indentation for the egg. Be careful not to scoop all the way through the mushroom. Discard the scrapings.

3 Brush the mushrooms with the remaining 2 tablespoons oil. Place the mushroom caps, stem sides down, on the prepared baking sheet. Roast, uncovered, alongside the vegetables for 15 minutes, or until the mushrooms are just tender. Turn the mushrooms stem sides up.

4 Reduce the oven temperature to 350°F. Crack one egg into each of the mushroom caps. Sprinkle lightly with salt and black pepper. Bake, uncovered, for 8 to 10 minutes, or until the egg whites are completely set and the egg yolks are cooked to the desired doneness.

<u>5</u> While the eggs are baking, transfer the roasted tomato mixture to a medium bowl. Mash to the desired consistency using a potato masher; add a small amount of water, if needed. (Or use a blender to blend to a chunky sauce.) Stir in the olives, oregano, and vinegar. Season to taste with additional salt and black pepper.

<u>6</u> To serve, spoon some of the sauce onto each of two serving plates. Top the sauce with the egg-stuffed mushrooms. Spoon the remaining sauce on top of the mushrooms. Sprinkle with basil.

Protein: 11 g • **Net Carbs:** 14 g • **Fat:** 36 g

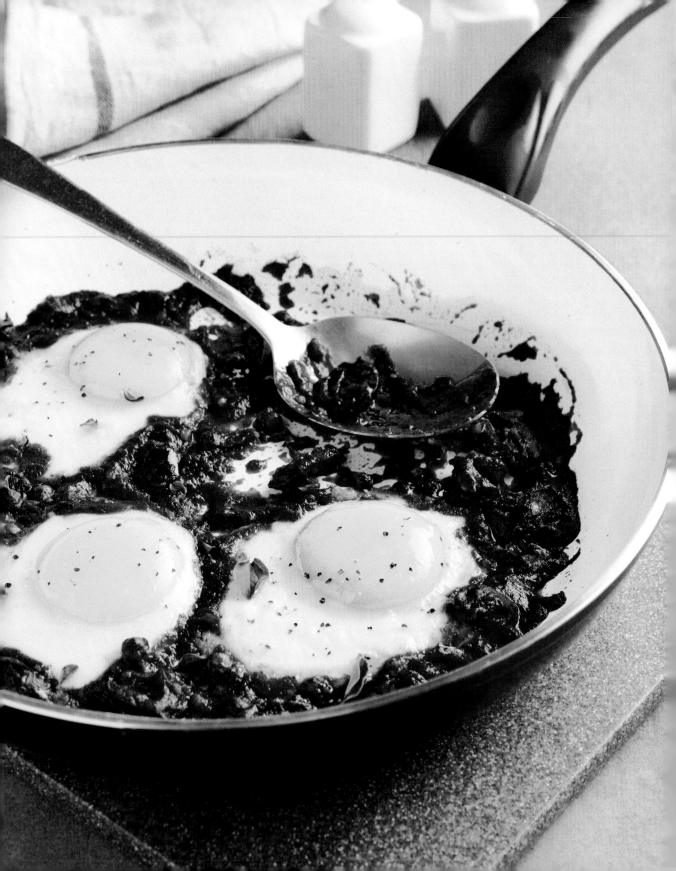

poached eggs over tomato-olive-caper sauce with fresh oregano

VEGETARIAN

START TO FINISH: 25 minutes

SERVES 2

3 tablespoons olive oil

1 tablespoon minced garlic

1¼ cups salt-free tomato *passata* (puréed, strained tomatoes)

8 pitted kalamata olives, halved

1 tablespoon capers, rinsed and drained

1 tablespoon minced fresh oregano leaves

⅛ teaspoon freshly ground black pepper

4 large eggs

Sea salt

1 Heat the oil in a deep, medium skillet over medium-high heat. When hot, add the garlic and sauté for 2 minutes (do not let it brown). Add the tomatoes, olives, capers, oregano, and pepper and bring to a boil over high heat. Boil until the sauce reduces to about 1 cup and has thickened, about 5 minutes.

2 Crack an egg into a ramekin and then add it to the sauce. Repeat rapidly with the remaining eggs and sprinkle the eggs evenly with salt.

3 Cover the pan and reduce the heat to medium-low. Simmer until the whites are opaque and the yolks are firm around the edges but still molten in the center, 3 to 5 minutes. Serve immediately.

Protein: 16 g • **Net Carbs:** 14 g • **Fat:** 34 g

vegetable hash with fried eggs

VEGETARIAN

START TO FINISH: 20 minutes

SERVES 2

4 tablespoons ghee

½ cup coarsely chopped red bell pepper

¼ cup chopped onion

Dash of red pepper flakes

2 cups coarsely chopped broccoli florets

½ cup coarsely chopped zucchini

⅛ teaspoon salt

⅛ teaspoon dried thyme

4 large eggs

¼ cup soft fresh vegan cheese, crumbled

2 teaspoons chopped fresh flat-leaf parsley

1 In a large skillet, heat 3 tablespoons ghee over medium-high heat. Add the bell pepper, onion, and red pepper flakes. Cook for 3 minutes, stirring occasionally. Add the broccoli, zucchini, salt, and thyme. Cook, stirring occasionally, for 5 to 6 minutes more, or until the vegetables are crisp-tender. Divide the vegetable mixture between two serving bowls.

2 In the same skillet, heat the remaining 1 tablespoon ghee over medium heat. Break the eggs into the skillet. Reduce the heat to low; cook the eggs for 3 to 4 minutes, or until the whites are completely set and the yolks start to thicken. Turn the eggs and cook for 30 seconds more for over-easy fried eggs.

3 Serve the fried eggs over the vegetable hash. Top with cheese and sprinkle with parsley.

Protein: 18 g • **Net Carbs:** 9 g • **Fat:** 44 g

salads and sides

Let's be honest, salads can be freaking boring sometimes. Not here. These Keto-tarian salads are simply delicious, if I do say so myself. The sides are a great way to add more colors of the plant-based rainbow to your day. "Eat your veggies" never tasted so good.

cucumber, radish, and snap pea salad

VEGAN, VEGETARIAN, AIP

START TO FINISH: 10 minutes

SERVES 2

3 tablespoons avocado oil

1 tablespoon white wine vinegar

2 teaspoons coconut aminos

1 cup sliced English cucumber

½ cup fresh sugar snap peas, sliced crosswise

¼ cup thinly sliced radish

1 medium avocado, halved, pitted, peeled, and cubed

½ large sheet toasted nori, cut into matchsticks

1 teaspoon toasted sesame seeds (optional)

1 In a medium bowl, whisk together the oil, vinegar, and coconut aminos. Add the cucumber, sugar snap peas, and radish; toss to coat.

2 Gently stir in the avocado. Top with nori and sesame seeds, if using.

Protein: 2 g • **Net Carbs:** 4 g • **Fat:** 31 g

NOTE: For an AIP-compliant recipe, do not use the sesame seeds.

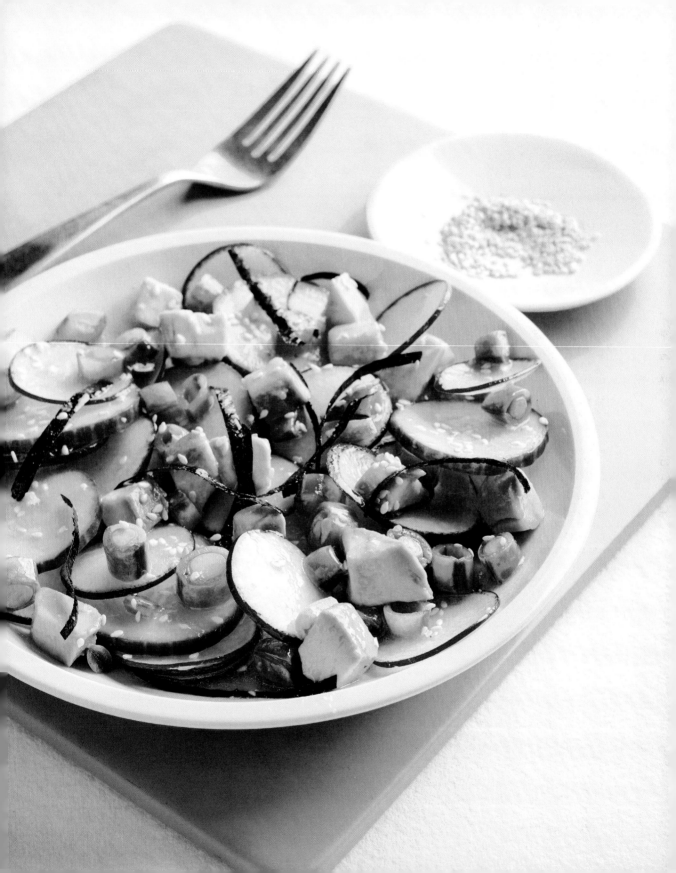

apple cider broccoli salad

VEGETARIAN

PREP: 5 minutes
COOK: 5 minutes

SERVES 2

¼ cup organic apple cider vinegar

2 tablespoons chopped raspberries

½ teaspoon fennel seeds, toasted

½ teaspoon bee pollen

¼ cup extra virgin olive oil

2 cups broccoli florets, blanched

¼ red onion, diced

¼ cup thinly sliced red cabbage

1 small carrot, peeled and thinly sliced

2 green onions (scallions), sliced

1 garlic clove, minced

Salt and freshly ground black pepper

1 In a small saucepan, combine the vinegar, raspberries, fennel seeds, and bee pollen. Bring to a boil; reduce the heat to low and simmer until reduced by half. Allow to cool for 5 minutes, then slowly whisk in the oil.

2 In a large bowl, mix together the broccoli, onion, cabbage, carrot, green onions, and garlic. Toss with the dressing. Season with salt and pepper.

Protein: 4 g • **Net Carbs:** 9 g • **Fat:** 28 g

sesame-lemon fennel-cucumber slaw

VEGAN, VEGETARIAN

START TO FINISH: 15 minutes

SERVES 2

1 medium fennel bulb

¾ cup coarsely shredded English cucumber (about ½ cucumber)

4 medium radishes, very thinly sliced

1 green onion (scallion), thinly sliced

2 tablespoons fresh lemon juice

3 tablespoons toasted sesame oil

1 teaspoon toasted white sesame seeds

1 teaspoon toasted black sesame seeds

¼ teaspoon coarse salt

⅛ teaspoon red pepper flakes (optional)

¼ cup chopped fresh mint or cilantro

1 Trim the tops off the fennel bulb, reserving some of the feathery tops (fronds) for garnish. Trim a thin slice off the base of the bulb. Cut the bulb in half and cut out the core. Cut the remaining fennel bulb into very thin strips. In a medium bowl, combine the fennel, cucumber, radishes, and green onion.

2 In a small bowl, whisk together the juice, oil, sesame seeds, salt, and red pepper flakes, if using. Pour the dressing over the fennel mixture; toss to coat. Stir in the mint. Sprinkle with fennel fronds.

Protein: 2 g • **Net Carbs:** 8 g • **Fat:** 22 g

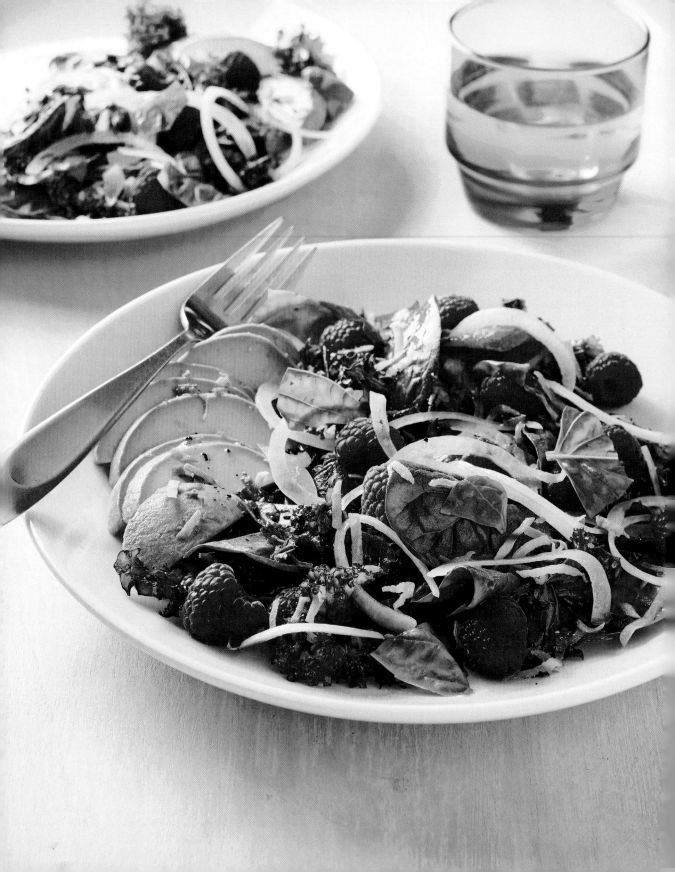

raspberry super salad with toasted coconut

VEGAN, VEGETARIAN, AIP

PREP: 20 minutes
STAND: 1 to 2 hours

SERVES 2

⅓ cup thin slivers Vidalia onion

3 tablespoons fresh lime juice

1 cup trimmed, torn fresh kale leaves

2 tablespoons olive oil

¼ teaspoon coarse salt

¼ teaspoon freshly ground black pepper

1 cup fresh baby spinach leaves

1 small avocado, halved, pitted, peeled, and thinly sliced

½ cup fresh raspberries

¼ cup large flaked coconut, toasted

¼ cup torn fresh basil leaves

1 In a small bowl, combine the onion and juice; toss to coat. Press down on the onion to submerge it as much as possible. Cover; let stand for at least 1 hour or up to 24 hours (refrigerate if standing for more than 1 hour).

2 Meanwhile, in a medium bowl, combine the kale, 1 tablespoon oil, and ⅛ teaspoon salt. Using clean fingers, gently massage and mix the kale leaves with the oil mixture until the kale has wilted slightly. If needed, cover and chill 1 to 2 hours before serving.

3 Drain the onion, reserving 1 tablespoon of the soaking juice. In a small bowl, combine the reserved soaking juice, the remaining 1 tablespoon oil, the remaining ⅛ teaspoon salt, and the pepper.

4 To serve, toss the spinach with the kale in a bowl. Divide the kale mixture between two serving plates. Top evenly with the onion, avocado, raspberries, coconut, and basil. Drizzle with the dressing.

Protein: 4 g • **Net Carbs:** 9 g • **Fat:** 28 g

warm german brussels sprout salad

VEGAN, VEGETARIAN

START TO FINISH: 20 minutes

SERVES 2

¼ cup coconut oil

½ pound Brussels sprouts, stems removed, washed, dried, trimmed, and thinly sliced

1 small shallot, minced (2 tablespoons)

½ teaspoon caraway seeds

1 tablespoon no-sugar-added whole-grain mustard

½ teaspoon chopped currants

¼ cup sauerkraut, drained

3 ounces baby arugula leaves

¼ teaspoon kosher salt

½ teaspoon cracked black pepper

1 Heat the oil in a large skillet over medium heat. Add the Brussels sprouts and shallot and cook for 2 minutes, until the sprouts are warmed through but still crisp.

2 In a large bowl, combine the warm sprouts and shallots with the remaining ingredients and serve.

Protein: 5 g • **Net Carbs:** 8 g • **Fat:** 28 g

---

roasted cauliflower with hot sauce, olives, and lemon

VEGAN, VEGETARIAN

PREP: 5 minutes
ROAST: 35 minutes

SERVES 2

1 small head cauliflower, cut into 1-inch florets

3 tablespoons olive oil

1 teaspoon hot sauce

¼ teaspoon sea salt

⅓ cup pitted green olives, halved

1 teaspoon fresh lemon juice

½ teaspoon fresh lemon zest

1 Preheat the oven to 425°F. Line a rimmed baking dish with parchment paper or aluminum foil. In a medium bowl, toss the cauliflower with the oil, hot sauce, and salt. Pour onto the lined pan (reserve the bowl) and roast for 20 minutes.

2 Stir the cauliflower, add the olives to the pan, and continue roasting until the cauliflower is very tender and brown in spots, another 15 to 20 minutes. Pour the mixture into the bowl and toss with the juice and zest.

Protein: 3 g • **Net Carbs:** 5 g • **Fat:** 24 g

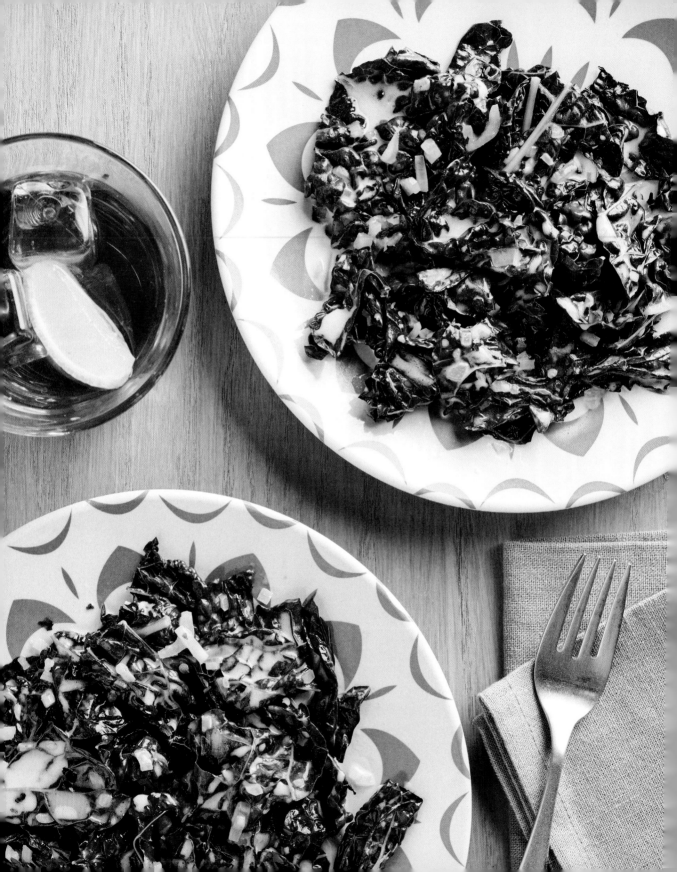

creamed kale

VEGAN, VEGETARIAN, AIP

PREP: 8 minutes
COOK: 6 minutes

SERVES 2

3 tablespoons coconut oil

3 tablespoons finely chopped shallots

½ teaspoon minced fresh ginger

5 cups chopped Tuscan kale leaves

⅛ teaspoon salt

½ cup full-fat coconut milk

2 teaspoons coconut aminos

1 In a large skillet, heat the oil over medium heat. Add the shallots and ginger; cook and stir for 1 minute, until fragrant. Add the kale and salt; cook and stir for 2 to 3 minutes or until the kale is just wilted.

2 Stir in the milk; cover and cook for 2 to 4 minutes, until the kale is tender. Stir in the coconut aminos and serve.

Protein: 8 g • **Net Carbs:** 13 g • **Fat:** 30 g

crispy brussels sprouts with fish sauce and lime

VEGAQUARIAN, AIP

PREP: 5 minutes
COOK: 20 minutes

SERVES 2

½ pound small Brussels sprouts, ends trimmed, halved

3 tablespoons olive oil

1 teaspoon fish sauce

Freshly ground black pepper

1 teaspoon fresh lime juice

½ teaspoon fresh lime zest

1 Preheat the oven to 400°F. Line a half-sheet pan with parchment paper. In a medium bowl, toss the sprouts with the oil, fish sauce, and pepper to taste. Pour onto the lined pan (reserve the bowl), arrange the sprouts cut side down, and roast for about 20 minutes, stirring halfway through the roasting time, until tender and very brown and crispy in spots.

2 Pour the sprouts into the bowl, toss with the juice and zest, and serve.

Protein: 4.5 g • **Net Carbs:** 7 g • **Fat:** 21 g

tangy green beans with olives

VEGAN, VEGETARIAN, AIP

PREP: 10 minutes
COOK: 10 minutes

SERVES 2

2 cups fresh green beans, trimmed (8 ounces)

2 tablespoons olive oil

¼ teaspoon coarse salt

¼ teaspoon freshly ground black pepper

¼ cup pitted kalamata olives, coarsely chopped

1 tablespoon white wine vinegar

2 tablespoons chopped fresh parsley

2 tablespoons coarsely grated fresh cauliflower (optional)

1 Place a steamer basket in a large skillet; add enough water to almost touch the bottom of the basket. Bring the water to a boil. Add the beans to the steamer basket. Cover and steam the beans for 6 to 8 minutes, or until crisp-tender. Remove the steamer basket of beans. Discard the water. Carefully wipe the skillet dry.

2 In the same skillet, heat the oil over medium-high heat. Add the beans, salt, and pepper. Cook, stirring occasionally, for 3 to 5 minutes, or until the beans are lightly browned. Remove from the heat.

3 Just before serving, toss the beans with the olives and vinegar. Divide the beans between two serving plates. Sprinkle with parsley and cauliflower, if using.

Protein: 2 g • **Net Carbs:** 6 g • **Fat:** 18 g

roasted broccoli with lemon and olives

VEGAN, VEGETARIAN, AIP

PREP: 5 minutes
ROAST: 30 minutes

SERVES 4

6 cups broccoli florets

4 tablespoons olive oil

¼ teaspoon salt

¼ cup pitted kalamata olives, chopped

½ teaspoon finely shredded fresh lemon zest

2 teaspoons fresh lemon juice

Lemon wedges, for garnish

1 Preheat the oven to 400°F.

2 Place the broccoli in a large bowl and drizzle with 3 tablespoons oil and the salt; mix well to coat. Spread evenly on a large rimmed baking sheet.

3 Roast for 20 minutes; stir. Roast for 10 to 15 minutes more, or until the broccoli is tender and browned. Transfer to a serving bowl.

4 In a small bowl, combine the olives, zest, juice, and the remaining 1 tablespoon oil. Spoon the olive mixture over the roasted broccoli and garnish with the lemon wedges.

Protein: 4 g • **Net Carbs:** 6 g • **Fat:** 16 g

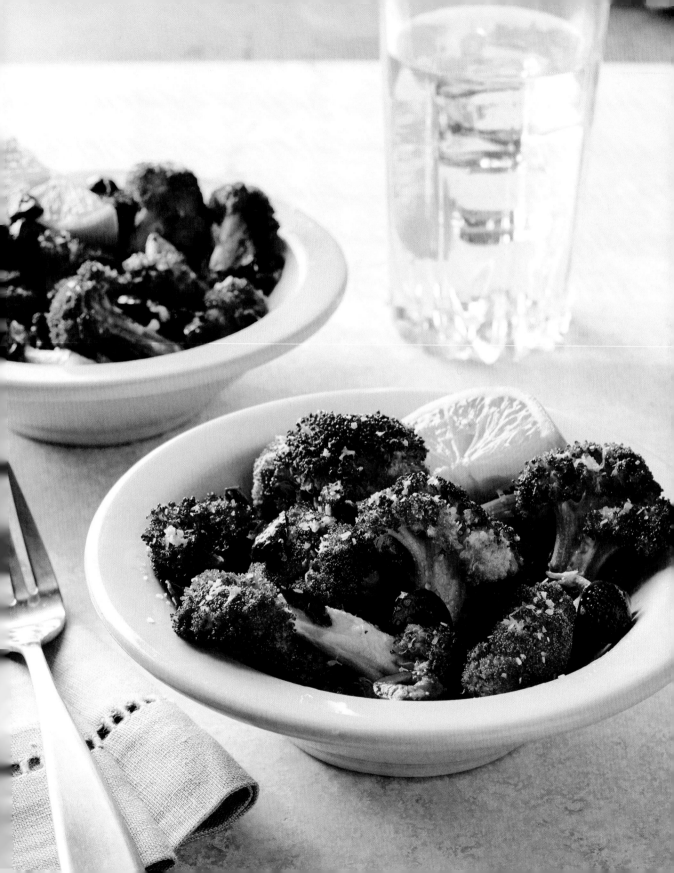

smoothies, elixirs, and snacks

I am a superfan of (and sucker for) superfood elixirs, smoothies, and snacks. These are some of my favorite keto treats and drinks in the cosmos. One of the many great things about going veggie and keto is that you don't *need* to snack just to get to the next meal. We have slain the hangry dragon and have achieved food freedom. There is no *need* here. The easy and delicious ideas in this section can be used whenever you like.

coconut-raspberry smoothie

VEGAN, VEGETARIAN, AIP

START TO FINISH: 5 minutes

SERVES 2

3 cups plain unsweetened coconut milk

1 cup fresh raspberries

¼ cup unsweetened shredded coconut

2 tablespoons coconut oil*

2 teaspoon vanilla extract

⅛ teaspoon sea salt

2 to 4 drops liquid stevia (optional)

Combine all of the ingredients in the container of a blender and purée on high speed until smooth, about 2 minutes. Serve immediately.

Protein: 1 g • **Net Carbs:** 6 g • **Fat:** 24 g

*NOTE: Because coconut oil is solid at room temperature, you'll get the smoothest texture in this drink if you use a high-powered blender to make it.

strawberry-avocado smoothie

VEGAN, VEGETARIAN

START TO FINISH: 5 minutes

SERVES 2

18 raw whole cashews, soaked overnight*

1 cup full-fat coconut milk

½ cup cold water

1 cup frozen sliced strawberries

½ medium avocado, halved, pitted, and peeled

2 tablespoons hemp protein powder

1 tablespoon avocado oil

4 to 6 drops liquid stevia

Combine the soaked cashews, milk, water, strawberries, avocado, hemp protein powder, and oil in the container of a blender. Cover and blend until smooth. Sweeten to taste with stevia.

Protein: 9 g • **Net Carbs:** 12 g • **Fat:** 34 g

*TIP: To soak the cashews, place in a small bowl and cover with cold water. Refrigerate overnight. Drain and rinse the cashews before using.

spirulina super smoothie

VEGAN, VEGETARIAN

START TO FINISH: 10 minutes

SERVES 2

½ cucumber, seeded (unpeeled)

½ large avocado, halved, pitted, peeled, and cubed

¼ cup raspberries

1½ cups coconut milk

1 ounce (about 1 cup) collard greens, stemmed and torn

2 tablespoons almond butter

1 teaspoon spirulina

1 teaspoon matcha powder

½ teaspoon fresh lemon juice (optional)

1 In the container of a blender, place the cucumber, avocado, and raspberries, followed by the remaining ingredients.

2 Blend in stages using the pulse function until the desired consistency is reached, scraping down the sides as necessary.

3 Enjoy immediately or refrigerate for up to 2 days. Some separation may naturally occur if allowed to sit.

Protein: 6 g • **Net Carbs:** 6 g • **Fat:** 18 g

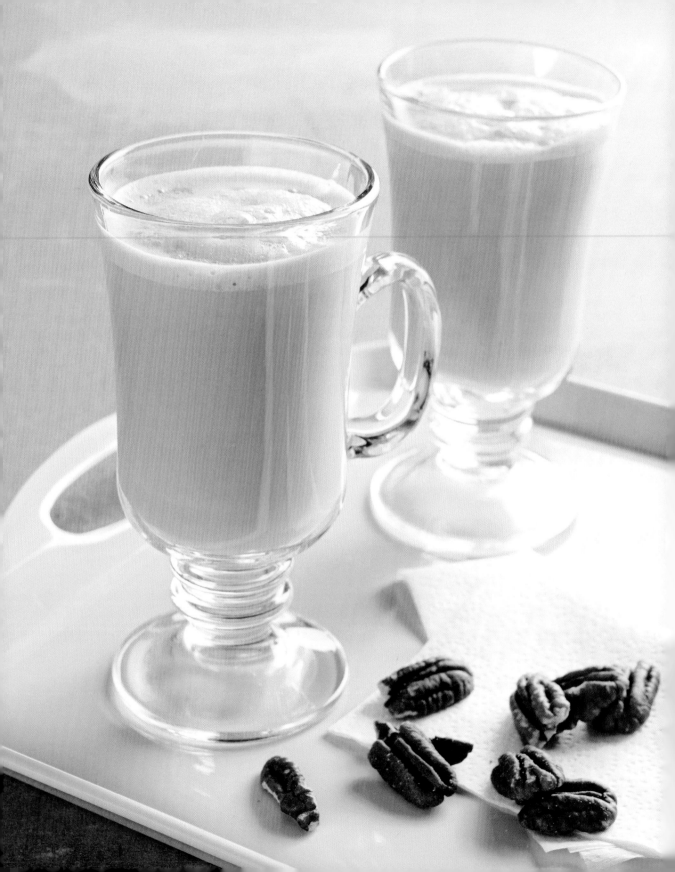

matcha latte

VEGAN, VEGETARIAN, AIP

START TO FINISH: 10 minutes

SERVES 1

½ cup full-fat coconut milk

1 teaspoon matcha powder

1 tablespoon virgin coconut oil

2 to 4 drops liquid stevia (optional)

In a small saucepan, combine the milk and ½ cup water. Heat over medium heat until hot and steamy but not boiling. Pour into the container of a heatproof blender; add the matcha powder and oil. Cover and blend until frothy. Sweeten to taste with stevia, if using. Pour into a mug and serve.

Protein: 3 g • **Net Carbs:** 2 g • **Fat:** 30 g

daily detox drink

VEGETARIAN, AIP

PREP: 5 minutes
STAND: 3 hours

SERVES 2

1 cup hot water

1 tablespoon diced fresh ginger

One 3-inch cinnamon stick, broken

2 teaspoons bee pollen

½ grapefruit, peeled and sectioned

1½ cups torn beet greens

2 sprigs fresh cilantro, stems trimmed

1 In a 2-cup glass measuring cup, combine the water, ginger, cinnamon, and bee pollen. Cover; let steep for 3 hours or overnight in the refrigerator. Strain the liquid through a fine sieve, discarding the solids.

2 Pour the liquid into the container of a blender. Add the grapefruit sections, beet greens, and cilantro. Blend until smooth. Serve over ice. Store any leftovers in the refrigerator.

Protein: 2 g • **Net Carbs:** 8 g • **Fat:** 1 g

TIP: Add 1 tablespoon of MCT oil or coconut oil if you want to increase your healthy fat.

fat bombs

COCOA ALMOND BUTTER FAT BOMBS

¼ cup virgin coconut oil

¼ cup almond butter

1 ounce unsweetened baking chocolate

1 tablespoon cocoa

½ teaspoon stevia drops

CHOCOLATE PEPPERMINT MACADAMIA NUT BOMBS

½ cup virgin coconut oil

½ cup cocoa

5 drops food-grade peppermint essential oil or extract

¼ cup finely chopped macadamia nuts

Pinch of sea salt

½ teaspoon stevia drops

COCONUT LEMON FAT BOMBS

½ cup virgin coconut oil

½ cup coconut butter

2 tablespoons lemon juice

1 tablespoon lemon zest

½ teaspoon stevia drops

1 Melt the ingredients in a pan over low heat. Stir continuously to avoid burning. You can also use a chocolate melter or double boiler.

2 Pour into silicone molds. Place in the freezer until hardened. Remove from the molds and store in a sealed container in the freezer.

Depending on size:

Protein: 2 g • **Net Carbs:** 2 g • **Fat:** 15 g

baked avocado fries
with smoky tomato mayo

VEGETARIAN

PREP: 10 minutes
COOK: 25 minutes

SERVES 2

¾ cup almond flour

¼ teaspoon chili powder

¼ teaspoon salt

2 tablespoons plain, unsweetened almond or cashew milk

1 large avocado, halved, pitted, peeled, and cut into 8 slices

¼ cup avocado-oil mayonnaise

1 teaspoon tomato paste

1 teaspoon fresh lime juice

Dash of smoked paprika

1 Preheat the oven to 400°F. Line a half-sheet pan with parchment paper and spray with olive oil cooking spray. In a small bowl, whisk together the flour, chili powder, and salt. Pour the milk into a small bowl.

2 One at a time, carefully dip each avocado slice in the flour, then the milk, and then again in the flour. Place the coated pieces on the pan. Spray both sides of the avocado slices evenly with olive oil cooking spray.

3 Bake until golden brown and crispy on the outside, turning over halfway through, for about 25 minutes total (do not let them burn).

4 While the fries bake, whisk together the mayonnaise, tomato paste, juice, and smoked paprika. Serve the hot fries with the mayonnaise.

Protein: 11 g • **Net Carbs:** 7 g • **Fat:** 57 g

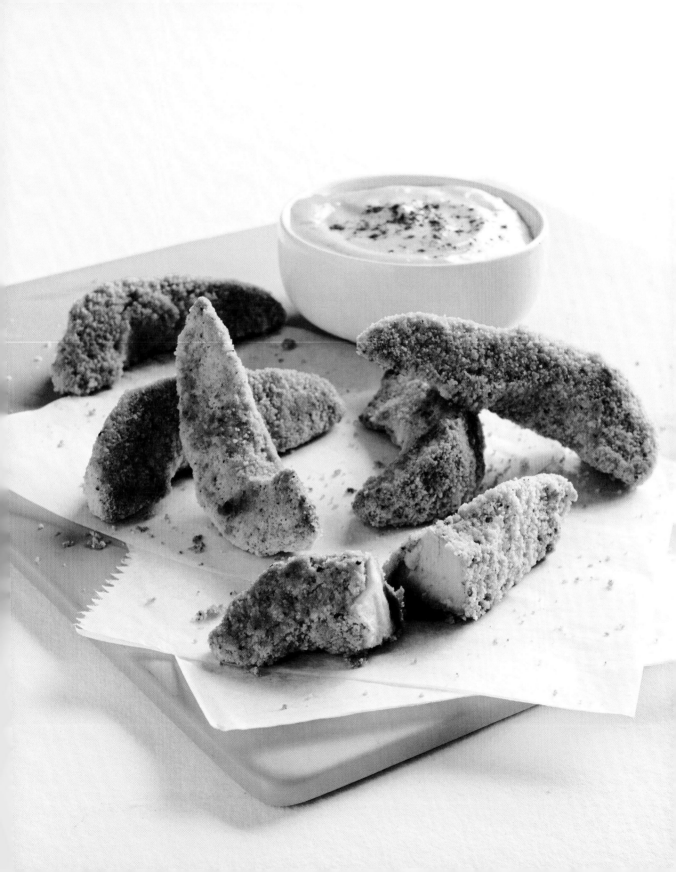

spiced coconut mixed nuts

VEGAN, VEGETARIAN

PREP: 10 minutes
BAKE: 12 minutes
COOL: 30 minutes

**MAKES ABOUT 2 CUPS
(6 SERVINGS)**

¾ cup raw almonds

½ cup raw macadamia nuts

½ cup shelled raw pistachio nuts

1 tablespoon refined coconut oil

½ teaspoon coarse salt

½ teaspoon ground coriander

½ teaspoon ground ginger

⅛ to ¼ teaspoon cayenne pepper

⅛ teaspoon ground cinnamon

⅓ cup unsweetened large flaked coconut

¼ cup shelled raw pumpkin seeds (pepitas)

1 Preheat the oven to 350°F. Spread the almonds, macadamia nuts, and pistachio nuts in a large shallow baking pan. Add the oil to the pan. In a small bowl, combine the salt, coriander, ginger, cayenne, and cinnamon. Sprinkle over the nuts. Bake for 2 minutes or until the oil is melted. Stir well to coat the nuts with the spices and oil.

2 Bake for 10 minutes more, stirring once. Add the flaked coconut and pumpkin seeds. Bake for 2 to 3 minutes more, or until the nuts and coconut are toasted. Cool in the pan on a wire rack. Store in an airtight container for up to 2 weeks.

Protein: 9 g • **Net Carbs:** 5 g • **Fat:** 29 g

kale chips with toasted sesame seeds, rice vinegar, lime, and sesame oil

VEGAN, VEGETARIAN

PREP: 5 minutes
BAKE: 30 minutes

SERVES 2

1 bunch fresh kale leaves, stems removed and leaves torn and patted dry (8 cups packed)

2 tablespoons avocado oil

2 tablespoons toasted sesame oil

4 teaspoons toasted sesame seeds

2 teaspoons unseasoned rice vinegar

1 teaspoon fresh lime zest

¼ teaspoon sea salt

1 Preheat the oven to 400°F. Line a half-sheet pan with parchment paper. In a large bowl, toss the kale with the oils and transfer to the pan (reserve the bowl). Bake until crisp, stirring halfway through, about 30 minutes.

2 Transfer the chips to the bowl. Add the sesame seeds, vinegar, zest, and salt and gently toss. Serve immediately.

Protein: 12 g • **Net Carbs:** 14 g • **Fat:** 32 g

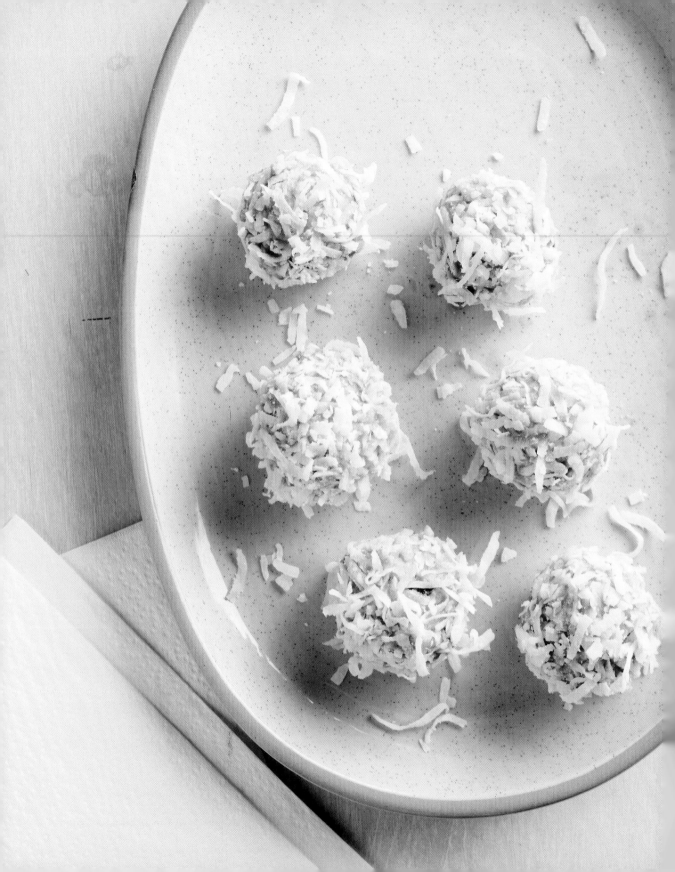

coconut-almond balls

VEGAN, VEGETARIAN

PREP: 10 minutes
CHILL: 40 minutes

SERVES 8

⅓ cup preservative-free, sugar-free creamy almond butter

¼ cup melted virgin coconut oil

1 tablespoon cacao nibs

¼ teaspoon vanilla

¼ cup finely shredded unsweetened coconut

1 In a medium bowl, combine the almond butter, oil, cacao nibs, and vanilla; mix well. Cover and refrigerate 30 to 40 minutes, or until firm enough to handle.

2 Place the coconut in a small dish. Using a 1-tablespoon measure, scoop the mixture into 8 portions and drop onto the coconut. Working quickly, roll into balls. Refrigerate for 10 minutes before eating. Store, covered, in the refrigerator.

Protein: 2 g • **Net Carbs:** 2 g • **Fat:** 14 g

TIP: Freeze for longer storage. Thaw slightly before eating.

fish and shellfish

Plant-centric + wild-caught fish = vegaquarian! Let's jump into the water and tap into the magic of the sea. These fresh dishes are the ketogenic-pescatarian ideas for those of you who want some more options in your Ketotarian plan. Our blue planet's most bioavailable sources of omega fats and trace minerals are found in these oceanic superfoods. You can bring these tasty seafood meals into the rotation whenever you like for a well-rounded, clean ketogenic approach.

lemon-garlic salmon with broccoli rabe

VEGAQUARIAN, AIP

PREP: 5 minutes
COOK: 10 minutes

SERVES 2

3 tablespoons olive oil

Two 6-ounce salmon fillets, skin on

1½ teaspoons fresh lemon juice

1 garlic clove, minced

¼ teaspoon salt

¼ teaspoon freshly ground black pepper

1 tablespoon coconut oil

½ pound broccoli rabe, thick stems removed, cut into 1-inch pieces

1½ teaspoons fresh lemon zest

1½ teaspoons capers, drained

2 tablespoons pitted kalamata olives, sliced

1 tablespoon chopped fresh dill

1 Preheat the broiler to high and position the upper rack 6 inches below the broiler. Brush a baking dish with 1 tablespoon olive oil. Lay the salmon in the dish, skin side down. Drizzle with the juice, the remaining 2 tablespoons olive oil, and garlic. Season with salt and pepper. Broil for 5 minutes, or until the salmon is cooked through.

2 Meanwhile, heat the coconut oil in a skillet over medium-high heat. Add the broccoli rabe and cook, stirring frequently, for 2 minutes. Remove from the heat. Stir in the zest, capers, olives, and dill.

3 Serve the salmon over the broccoli rabe mixture.

Protein: 38 g • **Net Carbs:** 1 g • **Fat:** 39 g

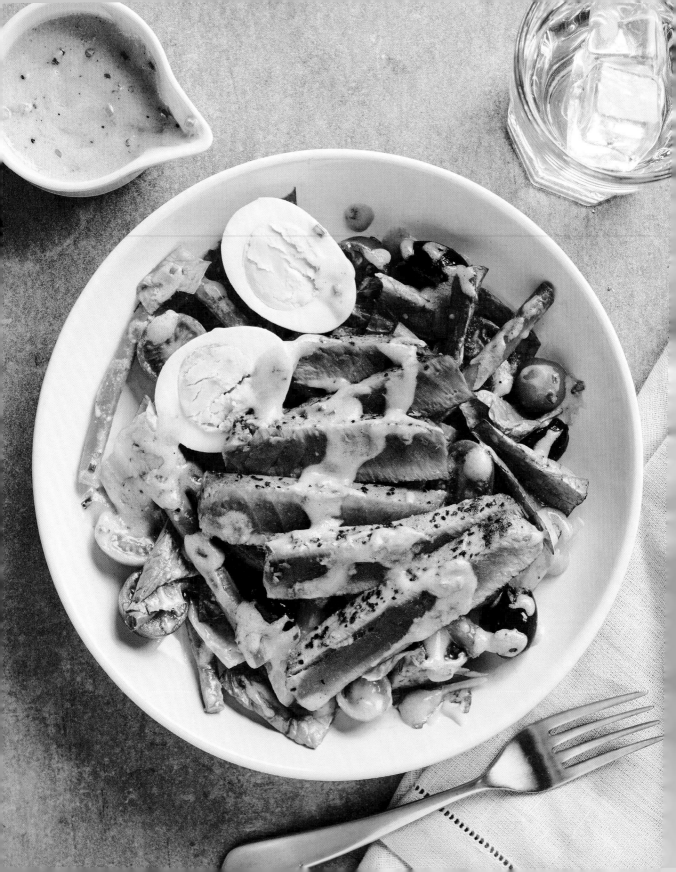

black pepper tuna niçoise salad with eggs, olives, and dijon vinaigrette

VEGAQUARIAN

PREP: 25 minutes
COOK: 20 minutes

SERVES 2

1 teaspoon salt

4 ounces slender fresh green beans, trimmed

4 large eggs

6 ounces raw sushi-grade tuna steak (1 to 2 inches thick), cut into two steaks

¼ teaspoon plus a dash of freshly ground black pepper

3 tablespoons avocado oil

2 tablespoons cider vinegar

1 teaspoon Dijon mustard

2 teaspoons minced fresh chives

2 cups chopped romaine leaves, rinsed and spun dry

8 cherry or grape tomatoes, halved

8 pitted oil-cured olives, such as niçoise

1 Fill a medium bowl with ice water and ½ teaspoon salt. Fill a small saucepan two-thirds full of water, add ¼ teaspoon salt, cover, and bring to a boil. Once boiling, stir in the green beans and boil until crisp-tender, but still bright green, about 4 minutes. Using a slotted spoon, transfer the beans to the ice water and swish around for a couple of minutes. (Leave the water boiling in the pot, and leave the ice water in the bowl.) Remove the beans with the slotted spoon.

2 Add the eggs to the boiling water and cook for exactly 10 minutes. Using the slotted spoon, transfer the eggs to the bowl of ice water and let sit for about 3 minutes. Remove the eggs from the ice water and peel them. Cut the eggs into halves vertically and set aside.

3 Pat both sides of the tuna dry with paper towels. Season both sides of both pieces evenly with a ¼ teaspoon salt and ¼ teaspoon pepper.

4 Heat 1 tablespoon oil in an 8-inch nonstick sauté pan over medium-high heat. Once hot, add the tuna and sear until golden on one side, about 2 minutes. Flip and cook until the other side is similarly golden but the insides are still bright

recipe continues

pink, 1 to 2 minutes more. Transfer the tuna to a cutting board and cut it on the bias against the grain into thin slices.

5 Meanwhile, in a small bowl, whisk together the remaining 2 tablespoons oil, vinegar, mustard, chives, the remaining ¼ teaspoon salt, and a dash of pepper.

6 In a medium bowl, combine the beans, romaine, tomatoes, olives, and three-quarters of the vinaigrette. Toss gently with tongs and divide between two dinner plates. To each plate, add the egg and tuna slices. Drizzle the egg and tuna slices evenly with the remaining vinaigrette and serve immediately.

Protein: 36 g • **Net Carbs:** 7 g • **Fat:** 34 g

NOTE: For an AIP-compliant recipe, omit the eggs.

albacore tuna salad with grapefruit and avocado

VEGAQUARIAN, AIP

START TO FINISH: 15 minutes

SERVES 2

One 12-ounce can wild albacore tuna, drained

¼ cup avocado-oil mayonnaise

2 tablespoons minced shallot or red onion

2 teaspoons fresh lime juice

1 teaspoon fresh lime zest

⅛ teaspoon plus a dash of sea salt

⅛ teaspoon freshly ground black pepper

1 pink grapefruit, cut into sections

1 large avocado, halved. pitted, peeled, and sliced

1 In a medium bowl, stir together the tuna, mayonnaise, shallot, 1 teaspoon juice, zest, ⅛ teaspoon salt, and pepper.

2 Divide the grapefruit and avocado slices between two plates. Drizzle the avocado with the remaining 1 teaspoon juice and season the grapefruit and avocado with a dash of salt. Top with the tuna salad.

Protein: 47 g • **Net Carbs:** 14 g • **Fat:** 37 g

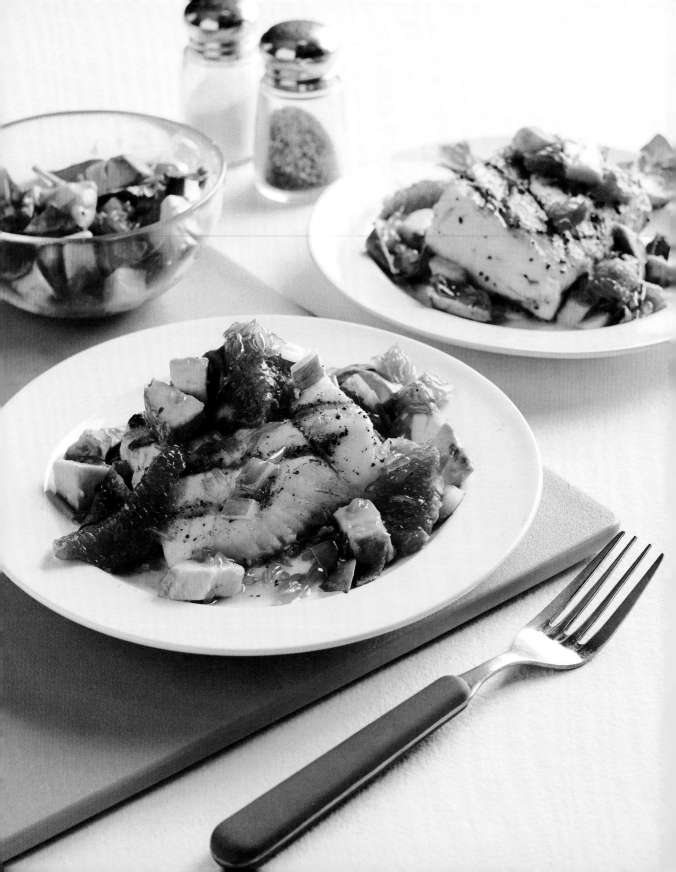

grilled halibut with grapefruit salsa

VEGAQUARIAN, AIP

PREP: 8 minutes
COOK: 10 minutes

SERVES 2

Two 4-to-5-ounce fresh or frozen halibut steaks, about 1 inch thick

¼ teaspoon ground coriander

¼ teaspoon coarse salt

¼ teaspoon ground ginger

¼ teaspoon freshly ground black pepper

2 tablespoons avocado oil or olive oil

1 tablespoon white wine vinegar

1 medium avocado, halved, pitted, peeled, and chopped

1 small grapefruit, peeled, seeded, and sectioned

2 tablespoons finely chopped red onion

1 cup torn fresh baby spinach leaves

⅓ cup coarsely chopped fresh basil leaves or flat-leaf parsley

1 Thaw the fish, if frozen. Rinse the fish with cold water and pat it dry with paper towels. In a small bowl, combine the coriander, salt, ginger, and ⅛ teaspoon pepper. Brush both sides of the fish with 1 tablespoon oil. Sprinkle the seasoning evenly over both sides of the fish.

2 For a charcoal grill, place the fish on the rack of an uncovered grill directly over medium coals. Grill, turning once halfway through grilling, for 8 to 12 minutes, or until the fish begins to flake when tested with a fork. (For a gas grill, preheat the grill. Reduce the heat to medium. Place the fish on the grill rack over the heat. Cover and grill as directed.)

3 Meanwhile, in a medium bowl, whisk together the remaining 1 tablespoon oil, the vinegar, and the remaining ⅛ teaspoon pepper. Add the avocado, grapefruit, and onion; toss gently to combine. Right before serving, add the spinach and basil; toss gently to coat.

4 Serve the fish on top of the avocado mixture.

Protein: 24 g • **Net Carbs:** 11 g • **Fat:** 26 g

catfish po'boy wraps with celery root slaw

VEGAQUARIAN

PREP: 15 minutes
COOK: 10 minutes

SERVES 2

8 ounces fresh or frozen skinned catfish fillets

¾ cup coarsely shredded, trimmed, and peeled celery root or kohlrabi

⅓ cup chopped red bell pepper

1 green onion (scallion), thinly sliced

2 tablespoons avocado-oil mayonnaise

1 tablespoon fresh lemon juice

1 garlic clove, minced

½ teaspoon coarse salt

⅜ teaspoon freshly ground black pepper

⅓ cup almond meal

½ teaspoon paprika

¼ teaspoon ground mustard

1 large egg

¼ cup refined coconut oil or avocado oil

4 collard leaves, trimmed*

Lemon wedges (optional)

1 Thaw the fish, if frozen. Rinse the fish with cold water and pat it dry with paper towels. Cut the fillets into 4 even-sized portions; set aside. In a medium bowl, toss together the celery root, bell pepper, and green onion. In a small bowl, whisk together the mayonnaise, juice, garlic, ¼ teaspoon salt, and ⅛ teaspoon black pepper. Pour the dressing over the celery root mixture; toss to coat. Cover; chill while cooking the fish.

2 In a shallow dish, combine the almond meal, paprika, mustard, the remaining ¼ teaspoon salt, and the remaining ¼ teaspoon black pepper. In another shallow dish, beat the egg with a fork. Dip the fish pieces in the egg, turning to coat both sides. Allow the excess to drip off. Dip the fish in the almond mixture, turning to coat both sides.

3 In a large skillet, heat the oil over medium heat. Add the fish to the skillet. Cook, turning the fish once halfway through cooking, for 6 to 8 minutes, or until the fish is golden brown and flakes easily when tested with a fork.

<u>4</u> To serve, spoon the celery root slaw evenly over the collard leaves. Top the slaw with the fish. If desired, squeeze additional lemon juice over all. Fold the collard leaves up around the fish and slaw to eat.

Protein: 29 g • **Net Carbs:** 10 g • **Fat:** 55 g

---

*TIP: To make the collard leaves more pliable to wrap around the fish and slaw, add water to a skillet to make it three-fourths full. Bring to a boil. Add two collard leaves; cook for 1 to 2 minutes or until the leaves turn bright green and are more pliable. Carefully remove the leaves from the water; drain on paper towels. Repeat with the remaining leaves.

smoked trout lettuce wraps

VEGAQUARIAN

START TO FINISH: 10 minutes

SERVES 2

¼ cup avocado-oil mayonnaise

½ teaspoon finely shredded fresh lemon zest

1 teaspoon fresh lemon juice

1 teaspoon chopped fresh dill

6 butterhead or Bibb lettuce leaves

1 medium avocado, halved, pitted, peeled, and sliced

4 ounces flaked smoked trout

1 tablespoon chopped red onion

1 In a small bowl, stir together the mayonnaise, zest, juice, and dill. Set aside.

2 Place the lettuce leaves on a work surface. Divide the avocado, trout, and onion between the lettuce leaves. Top with the mayonnaise mixture.

Protein: 14 g • **Net Carbs:** 2 g • **Fat:** 37 g

smoked herring collard wraps

VEGAQUARIAN

START TO FINISH: 15 minutes (plus 5 minutes if blanching greens)

SERVES 2

FOR THE SAUCE

¼ cup avocado-oil mayonnaise

½ teaspoon finely shredded fresh lemon zest

1 teaspoon fresh lemon juice

1 tablespoon chopped fresh flat-leaf parsley

FOR THE WRAP

2 large collard green leaves

1 medium avocado, halved, pitted, peeled, and mashed

2 teaspoons fresh lemon juice

⅛ teaspoon salt

Dash of freshly ground black pepper

One 6.7-ounce can all-natural smoked wild kippers (herring fillets), drained and flaked

½ cup thinly sliced English cucumber

¼ cup matchstick-cut radishes

1 In a small bowl, stir together the mayonnaise, zest, juice, and parsley. Refrigerate until ready to serve.

2 Remove and discard the stems from the collard leaves. Use a sharp knife to shave down the tough spine on the back side of each leaf. (This will make them easier to roll.)

3 Place the trimmed collard green leaves on a work surface, top side up. In a small bowl, stir together the avocado, juice, salt, and pepper. Spread the avocado mixture down the center third of each leaf; layer with the flaked fish, cucumber, and radishes. Wrap burrito-style; secure with toothpicks and cut each wrap in half. Serve the sauce with the collard wraps for dipping.

Protein: 22 g • **Net Carbs:** 3 g • **Fat:** 44 g

TIP: For more tender collard green leaves, blanch in boiling water for 15 to 30 seconds. Cool in ice water; drain and pat dry. Handle carefully so as not to tear the leaves.

plank-smoked ginger-coconut salmon

VEGAQUARIAN, AIP

PREP: 1 hour (includes marinating time)
GRILL: 20 minutes

SERVES 2

One 10-to-12-ounce fresh or frozen wild salmon fillet, with skin

⅓ cup full-fat coconut milk

1 tablespoon liquid aminos

1 tablespoon grated fresh ginger

½ teaspoon grated fresh turmeric or ¼ teaspoon ground turmeric

¼ teaspoon freshly ground black pepper, plus more to taste

¼ teaspoon salt

2 tablespoons olive oil

1 garlic clove, minced

3 cups torn fresh kale leaves

2 lemons

1 tablespoon chopped fresh chives

1 Thaw the fish, if frozen. Rinse the fish with cold water and pat it dry with paper towels. Set aside. In a medium bowl, whisk together the milk, liquid aminos, ginger, turmeric, ¼ teaspoon pepper, and ⅛ teaspoon salt. Add the fish; turn gently to coat. Cover; marinate in the refrigerator for 1 to 3 hours, turning the fish once halfway through marinating.

2 Meanwhile, in a medium bowl, whisk together 1 tablespoon oil, the garlic, and the remaining ⅛ teaspoon salt. Add the kale; drizzle with the remaining 1 tablespoon oil. Using clean fingers, gently massage and mix the kale with the oil mixture until the kale has wilted slightly. Cover; chill for 1 to 2 hours or until ready to serve.

3 While the salmon is marinating, place a 15 × 6½ × ⅜-inch untreated cedar plank in a large pan with shallow sides. Add enough water to cover the plank; weight the plank down with a bowl if needed. Let the plank soak for at least 1 hour before grilling.

4 Remove the salmon from the marinade, discarding the excess marinade. Place the salmon on the soaked plank, skin side down. Thinly slice 1 lemon. Place the lemon slices on top of the fish.

recipe continues

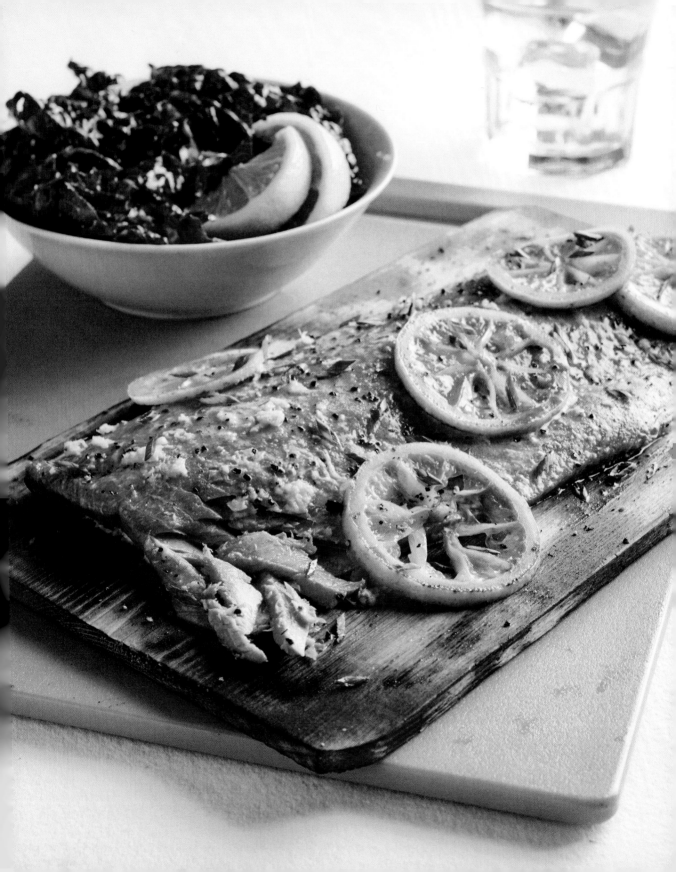

<u>5</u> For a charcoal grill, place the cedar plank with the salmon on the grill rack directly over medium coals. Cover and grill for 16 to 20 minutes, or just until the salmon begins to flake when tested with a fork. (For a gas grill, preheat the grill. Reduce the heat to medium. Place the cedar plank with the salmon on the grill rack over the heat. Grill as directed.)

<u>6</u> Meanwhile, cut the remaining lemon in half lengthwise. Use half to squeeze 1 tablespoon of juice. Add the juice to the kale salad; toss to coat. Cut the other half of the lemon into two wedges.

<u>7</u> Remove the salmon from the plank by using a large metal spatula to slide the salmon off the skin. Cut the salmon into two portions. Divide the salmon between two serving plates. Sprinkle with chives and pepper. Add the kale salad to the plates with the salmon. Serve with lemon wedges for squeezing over all.

Protein: 33 g • **Net Carbs:** 7 g • **Fat:** 26 g

salmon tacos

VEGAQUARIAN, AIP

PREP: 10 minutes
BAKE: 4 to 6 minutes
per ½-inch thickness

SERVES 2

FOR THE FILLING

8 ounces fresh skinless
salmon fillet

1 tablespoon olive oil

1½ teaspoons chili powder

¼ teaspoon ground cumin

¼ teaspoon salt

FOR THE SAUCE

¼ cup avocado-oil mayonnaise

½ teaspoon finely shredded
fresh lime zest

1 teaspoon fresh lime juice

1 tablespoon chopped fresh
cilantro

½ teaspoon minced fresh
jalapeño

FOR SERVING

2 tablespoons thinly sliced
radishes

6 butterhead or Bibb lettuce
leaves

Lime wedges

1 Preheat the oven to 450°F.

2 Rinse the fish and pat it dry with paper towels. Grease a shallow baking pan with avocado oil or olive oil and place the fish in the pan. Brush the fish with additional oil. Combine the chili powder, cumin, and salt in a small bowl. Sprinkle the seasoning blend evenly over the fish.

3 Bake, uncovered, for 4 to 6 minutes per ½-inch thickness of fish, or until the fish flakes easily when tested with a fork. Break the fish into bite-size chunks.

4 In a small bowl, combine the mayonnaise, zest, juice, cilantro, and jalapeño; mix well.

5 Serve the salmon and radishes in the lettuce leaves with the sauce and lime wedges.

Protein: 23 g • **Net Carbs:** 2 g • **Fat:** 38 g

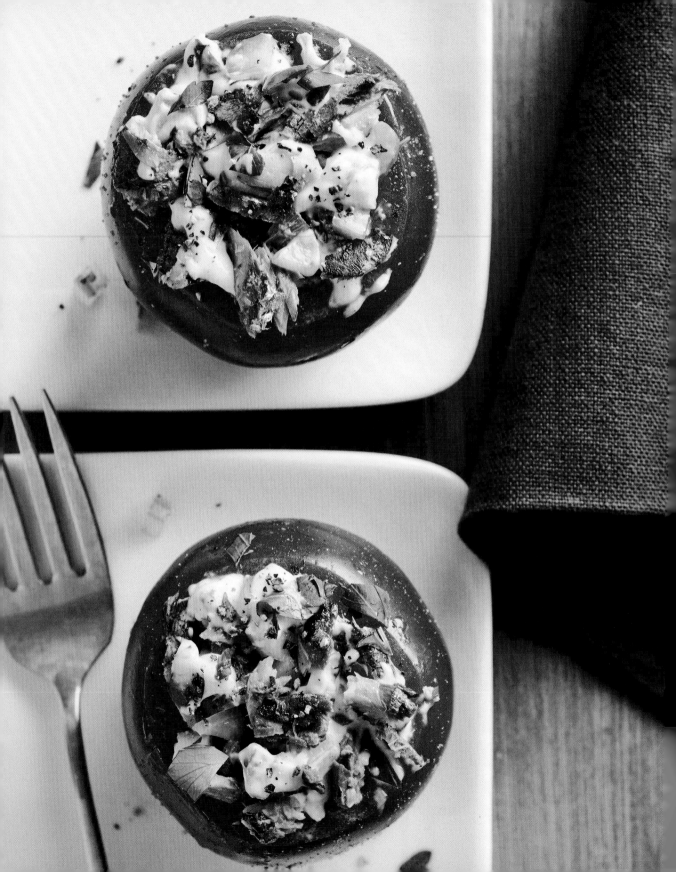

sardine-stuffed tomatoes

VEGAQUARIAN

START TO FINISH: 10 minutes

SERVES 2

2 medium ripe tomatoes

1 tablespoon extra virgin olive oil

1 teaspoon white wine vinegar

⅛ teaspoon salt

Dash of freshly ground black pepper

One 4.4-ounce can wild sardines in extra virgin olive oil, drained and flaked

¼ cup chopped celery

2 teaspoons chopped fresh flat-leaf parsley

3 tablespoons avocado-oil mayonnaise

1 teaspoon preservative-free, sugar-free Dijon mustard

1 Cut a thin slice off the top of each tomato. Scoop out and discard the pulp, leaving a shell. Drizzle the inside of the tomatoes with the oil and vinegar; sprinkle with salt and pepper.

2 In a medium bowl, combine the sardines, celery, parsley, mayonnaise, and mustard; mix well. Spoon into the tomatoes and serve.

Protein: 14 g • **Net Carbs:** 3 g • **Fat:** 39 g

italian eggplant and shrimp sauté

VEGAQUARIAN

PREP: 10 minutes
COOK: 15 minutes

SERVES 4

Sea salt

1 large eggplant, cut into
½-inch slices

2 tablespoons coconut oil

1 shallot, minced

2 garlic cloves, minced

½ pound wild-caught gulf
shrimp, peeled and deveined
(40–50 count)

¼ teaspoon sea salt

¼ teaspoon red pepper flakes

2 sun-dried tomatoes, chopped

2 tablespoons pitted kalamata
olives, coarsely chopped

¼ cup Basil Pesto (see recipe)

Lemon wedge

2 tablespoons chopped fresh
parsley

1 Lightly sprinkle salt on both sides of the eggplant slices. Lay the slices on a rack to allow the juices to extract, about 10 minutes. Pat dry and cut into 1-inch cubes.

2 Heat the oil in a large skillet over medium heat. Add the shallot and garlic. Cook for 2 minutes, until aromatic; move to the sides of the skillet.

3 Add the eggplant cubes to the skillet and cook for 3 minutes, stirring often.

4 Add the shrimp, salt, and red pepper flakes to the skillet. Cook until the shrimp are opaque, 3 to 5 minutes. Add the tomatoes, olives, and pesto. Heat through.

5 Squeeze with fresh lemon and sprinkle with parsley; serve immediately.

Protein: 12 g • **Net Carbs:** 9 g • **Fat:** 41 g

basil pesto

2 cups packed fresh basil leaves

1 cup packed fresh flat-leaf parsley

3 garlic cloves

½ cup pine nuts, toasted

1 cup extra virgin olive oil

½ teaspoon salt

¼ teaspoon freshly ground black pepper

In the container of a food processor, combine the basil, parsley, garlic, and pine nuts. Pulse until coarsely chopped. With the processor running, pour the oil in a thin stream into the container and blend until combined. Season with salt and pepper. Use immediately or freeze in desired portions for up to 3 months in tightly covered containers.

sautéed shrimp with white wine, garlic, chile, and olives

VEGAQUARIAN

PREP: 5 minutes

COOK: 8 minutes

SERVES 2

2 tablespoons olive oil

1 tablespoon minced fresh garlic

⅛ teaspoon red pepper flakes

10 ounces wild-caught shrimp, peeled and deveined (tails left on) (28–32 count)

¼ teaspoon Italian seasoning

¼ teaspoon sea salt

2 tablespoons dry white wine

10 pitted kalamata olives, halved

½ teaspoon fresh lemon zest

1 Heat the oil in a 10-inch nonstick skillet over medium-high heat. When hot, add the garlic and red pepper flakes and stir for 2 minutes (do not let it brown).

2 Add the shrimp, Italian seasoning, and salt and sauté for 2 minutes, until the shrimp just begins to turn opaque.

3 Stir in the wine and olives and continue sautéing just until the shrimp turns light pink (do not overcook), about 2 minutes more. Stir in the zest and serve immediately.

Protein: 20 g • **Net Carbs:** 4 g • **Fat:** 19 g

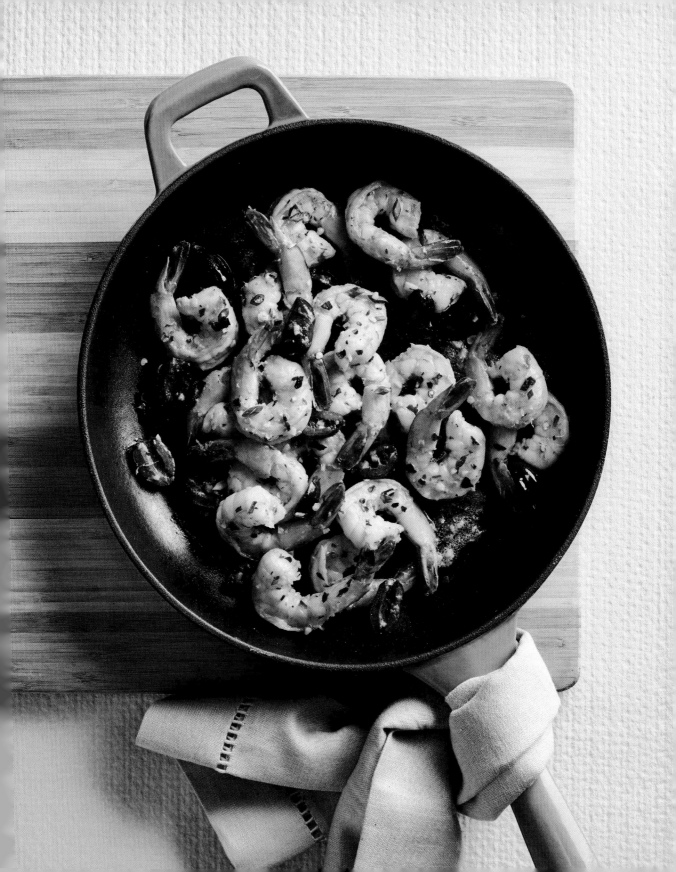

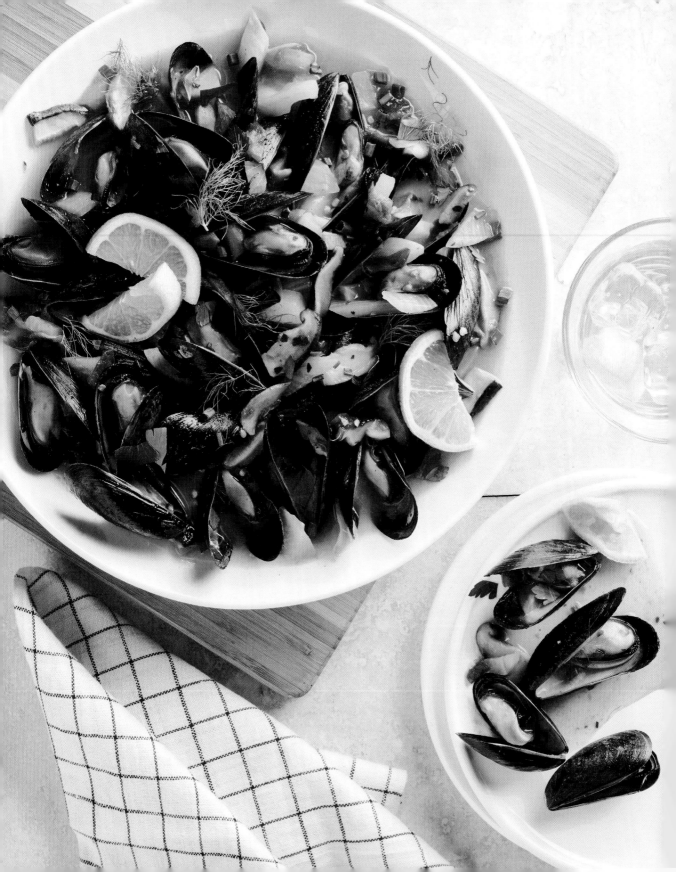

tomato-fennel broth bowls with mussels

VEGAQUARIAN

START TO FINISH: 45 minutes

SERVES 2

¼ cup sesame oil

1 small yellow onion, coarsely chopped

1 celery stalk, quartered

2 garlic cloves, crushed

One 3 × 3-inch piece dried kombu

3 thin slices fresh ginger

1 pound fresh mussels, in their shells

1 medium fennel bulb

¾ cup stemmed shiitake mushrooms, thinly sliced

⅓ cup dry white wine

1 cup chopped fresh tomatoes

2 teaspoons finely chopped fresh ginger

⅛ to ¼ teaspoon red pepper flakes

1 tablespoon chopped fresh chives

1 tablespoon chopped fresh flat-leaf parsley

1 In a 4-to-6-quart pot, heat 1 tablespoon oil over medium-high heat. Add the onion, celery, and garlic and cook, stirring occasionally, for 5 to 7 minutes, or until the vegetables are browned. Carefully add 2 cups water and the kombu and sliced ginger. Bring to a boil. Reduce the heat to low and simmer, covered, for 45 minutes.

2 Meanwhile, clean the mussels by rinsing them under cool running water and scrubbing them with a hard-bristle brush. Remove and discard the beards. Set the mussels aside.

3 Strain the stock through a fine strainer, reserving the liquid. Reserve the kombu; discard the remaining vegetables. Chop the kombu. Set the stock and kombu aside.

4 Trim the tops off the fennel bulb, reserving some of the feathery tops (fronds) for garnish. Trim a thin slice off the base of the bulb. Cut the bulb in half and cut out the core. Chop the fennel bulb. In the same pot, heat the remaining 3 tablespoons oil over medium heat. Add the fennel and mushrooms. Cook for 6 to 8 minutes, or until the vegetables are tender and starting to turn brown. Carefully add the wine and cook until the wine is almost completely evaporated, 2 to 3 minutes.

recipe continues

<u>5</u> Add the strained stock, tomatoes, finely chopped ginger, and red pepper flakes to the fennel mixture. Bring to a boil. Add the mussels; stir to combine. Cover, reduce the heat to medium, and cook for 5 to 7 minutes, or until the mussels open. Using a slotted spoon, transfer the mussels to two shallow serving bowls. Discard any mussels that do not open. Add the kombu to the pot with the stock. Ladle the stock mixture from the pot evenly over the mussels. Sprinkle with the reserved fennel fronds, chives, and parsley and serve.

Protein: 17 g • **Net Carbs:** 15 g • **Fat:** 30 g

southwest grilled scallops

VEGAQUARIAN

PREP: 15 minutes
GRILL: 6 minutes

SERVES 2

FOR THE AVOCADO SALSA

1 large avocado, halved, pitted, peeled, and chopped

¼ cup chopped red onion

2 tablespoons diced cucumber (unpeeled)

1 Roma tomato, seeds removed, diced

1½ teaspoons chopped fresh cilantro

1½ teaspoons fresh lime juice

½ teaspoon ground cumin

FOR THE SCALLOPS

6 sea scallops

1 tablespoon olive oil

½ teaspoon ground cumin

½ teaspoon dried oregano

¼ teaspoon cayenne pepper

1 For the salsa, in a medium bowl combine all of the salsa ingredients. Gently stir to combine.

2 For the scallops, heat the grill to medium-high. Prepare two 10-to-12-inch skewers; if using bamboo skewers, soak them in water for at least 30 minutes. Divide the scallops between the skewers. Drizzle with the oil. In a small bowl, combine the cumin, oregano, and cayenne. Sprinkle over the scallops.

3 Grill the scallops until firm, about 3 minutes per side. Remove to a plate and serve with the avocado salsa.

Protein: 17 g • **Net Carbs:** 9 g • **Fat:** 18 g

instant pot

People love their Instant Pots in a big way. If you don't know, Instant Pot is a multipurpose appliance that serves as a slow cooker, electric pressure cooker, steam cooker, yogurt maker, sauté pan, and warmer all in one. Basically, the Instant Pot is one multitalented little machine, and a great time-saver too. If you want to spend less time in the kitchen or want more convenient ideas, try delicious Ketotarian dishes in your Instant Pot (or similar kitchen tools).

creamy garlic dipping sauce

VEGETARIAN

PREP TIME: 5 minutes
COOK TIME: 5 minutes

MAKES ½ CUP

2 tablespoons ghee, plus more for the skillet

1 teaspoon minced fresh garlic

1 medium shallot, finely chopped

¼ cup full-fat coconut milk

Juice of 1 lemon

1 tablespoon chopped fresh thyme

Salt and freshly ground black pepper to taste

1 Heat a small amount of ghee in a small skillet over low heat. Add the garlic and shallot and cook until soft, 3 to 5 minutes. Remove from the heat and add 2 tablespoons ghee and the milk. Stir until well combined.

2 Heat over low heat until the sauce is warmed through and slightly bubbles. Remove from the heat and add the juice, thyme, salt, and pepper. Serve alongside the artichokes (see page 270).

Protein: 2 g • **Net Carbs:** 12 g • **Fat:** 21 g

instant pot artichokes

VEGAN, VEGETARIAN

PREP: 5 minutes
COOK: 10 minutes

SERVES 2

2 artichokes, 6 to 8 ounces each

1 small lemon

1 Rinse the artichokes and remove any damaged or bruised or inedible leaves. Next, trim the stems off the artichokes and cut the top third off. If this leaves any petals untrimmed, use kitchen scissors to cut the tops of them off. Throw away the stems and petal tops as they are not usable.

2 Cut the lemon in half. Reserve half and thinly slice the other half.

3 Pour 1 cup water into the Instant Pot. Place the sliced lemon in the water. Place the steamer basket in the Instant Pot and put the artichokes in the basket.

4 Take the other half of the lemon and use a hand juicer (or just your hand) to squeeze the juice over the top of the cut petals and top of the artichokes.

5 Close the pot and lock the lid.

6 Set the Instant Pot to Manual on high pressure.

7 Cooking time will be 8 to 10 minutes depending on the size of the artichokes, or 15 minutes if they are larger.

8 While the artichokes are cooking, prepare the Creamy Garlic Dipping Sauce (see recipe on page 269).

<u>9</u> Carefully open the pressure release valve after the time is up.

<u>10</u> Once the steam has dissipated, you can remove the lid and carefully remove the artichokes with a pair of tongs.

<u>11</u> Serve the artichokes warm with the dipping sauce.

Protein: 9 g • Net carbs: 23 g • **Fat:** 1 g

instant pot asparagus

VEGAN, VEGETARIAN

PREP: 5 minutes
COOK: 2 minutes

SERVES 4

1 pound fresh asparagus

1 tablespoon chopped fresh parsley

1 tablespoon chopped fresh chives

1 tablespoon onion powder

2 tablespoons olive oil

Salt and freshly ground black pepper

1 Cut 1 inch off the hard ends of the asparagus. Pour 1 cup water into the Instant Pot. Place the steamer basket in the Instant Pot. Place the asparagus in the basket and sprinkle it with the parsley, chives, and onion powder.

2 Close the pot and lock the lid.

3 Set the Instant Pot to Steamer. Set the timer for 2 minutes.

4 Carefully open the pressure release valve when the 2 minutes are up. When the steam has dissipated, you can remove the lid.

5 Place the asparagus in a serving dish, drizzle with oil, and sprinkle with salt and pepper to taste.

Protein: 3 g • **Net Carbs:** 4 g • **Fat:** 7 g

NOTE: This recipe can be converted for a slow cooker: Trim the asparagus as directed, but reduce the water to ¼ cup. Place the water in the bottom of the slow cooker, then spread the asparagus evenly across the bottom. Sprinkle with the seasonings and cook on high for 1 to 2 hours. The asparagus will lose some of its color but will still have all the taste! If your slow cooker is larger than 4 quarts, you may have to reduce the cooking time.

onion soup

VEGAN, VEGETARIAN

PREP: 5 minutes
COOK: 17 minutes

SERVES 5

4 tablespoons avocado oil

8 cups thinly sliced onions (a mix of yellow and sweet onions gives a nice balance)

1 garlic clove, minced

1 tablespoon red wine vinegar

6 cups preservative-free, sugar-free vegetable broth or stock

1 teaspoon sea salt

½ teaspoon freshly ground black pepper

1 teaspoon dried thyme

1 teaspoon dried oregano

½ teaspoon dried rosemary

½ teaspoon dried sage

NOTE: You can use a regular blender to blend the soup, but allow the soup to cool if you are unsure whether your blender tolerates high-temperature liquids. If your blender does handle high heat, use caution when transferring the liquid.

1 Set the Instant Pot to Sauté and add the avocado oil.

2 When the oil is hot, add the onions and garlic and cook, stirring occasionally, until they are translucent and slightly browned.

3 When the onions have reduced down, add the vinegar; stir and gently scrape to remove any pieces that may be stuck to the bottom.

4 Add the broth, salt, pepper, thyme, oregano, rosemary, and sage. Stir to combine.

5 Turn the Instant Pot off. Close the pot and lock the lid, making sure the vent is closed.

6 Set the Instant Pot to High Pressure and cook for 10 minutes.

7 Carefully open the pressure release valve after the time is up.

8 Use an immersion blender directly in the Instant Pot to blend the onion soup.

9 Ladle into individual dishes and serve warm.

Protein: 1 g • **Net Carbs:** 13 g • **Fat:** 11 g

Optional for added flavor boost
Drizzle with chive-infused olive oil or truffle oil.

creamy carrot soup

VEGAN, VEGETARIAN

PREP TIME: 10 minutes
COOK TIME: 15 minutes

SERVES 5

2 tablespoons avocado oil

2 cups chopped white onion

1½ pounds carrots, cut into ½-inch dice

1 celery stalk, chopped

2 garlic cloves, minced

1 teaspoon turmeric powder

2 teaspoons curry powder

½ teaspoon minced fresh ginger

½ teaspoon ground cumin

½ teaspoon sea salt

⅛ teaspoon freshly ground black pepper

5 cups preservative-free, sugar-free vegetable broth or stock

1 cup full-fat coconut milk

FOR GARNISH

Coconut cream

Toasted pumpkin seeds

Parsley

Fried sage

1 Set the Instant Pot to Sauté. Add the oil, onions, carrots, celery, and garlic and sauté for 5 to 7 minutes, until the onions soften and start to become translucent.

2 Add the turmeric, curry, ginger, cumin, salt, and pepper and mix for 30 seconds to 1 minute more.

3 Add the broth and milk and stir.

4 Close the pot and lock the lid. Set the Instant Pot to High Pressure and cook for 5 minutes. Carefully open the pressure release valve after the time is up.

5 Use an immersion blender directly in the Instant Pot to blend the carrot soup.

6 Ladle into individual serving dishes and serve warm. Garnish with toppings of your choice.

Protein: 1 g • **Net Carbs:** 6 g • **Fat:** 11 g

NOTE: You can use a regular blender to blend the soup, but allow the soup to cool if you are unsure whether your blender tolerates high-temperature liquids. If your blender does handle high heat, use caution when transferring the liquid.

coconut milk yogurt

VEGAN, VEGETARIAN

PREP: 10 minutes
COOK: 16 hours, 40 minutes

SERVES 6

Two 13.5-ounce cans full-fat coconut milk

1 tablespoon agar sea vegetable flakes (not powder)

1 teaspoon probiotic powder (dairy free)

1 In the Instant Pot, combine the milk and agar flakes. Set the Instant Pot to Sauté and bring the milk to a boil. Using a sterilized utensil, whisk the mixture so that the agar flakes dissolve as the milk boils.

2 Once the milk reaches a boil or at least 180°F, turn off the Instant Pot and stir until all of the flakes have dissolved.

3 Allow the mixture to cool to 110°F to 115°F to allow for fermentation (it will be warm to the touch without burning your finger).

4 When the milk has cooled, add the probiotic powder and mix well. Set the Instant Pot to Yogurt, then set the fermentation time to 10 to 24 hours (the longer the time, the tarter the yogurt will be).

5 Close the lid on the Instant Pot to help keep the yogurt at the correct temperature.

6 Once the yogurt has fermented, you can taste it to see if it needs more time for your preference. The texture of the yogurt will still be watery and separated, with a possible cream-colored film on top, which is normal. Pour the yogurt into a clean jar with a lid and place it in your refrigerator to set. Chilling the yogurt will allow it to thicken. Stir before serving.

Protein: 2 g • **Net Carbs:** 7 g • **Fat:** 22 g

meal plans

Now that you have seen how delicious going Ketotarian can be, let's put it all together and see what a day in the life of a Ketotarian looks like. I made these meal plans to be a guide, but feel free to personalize the recipes and plans by swapping foods in and out as you wish, keeping in mind any macro changes that may result. Of course, if you're incorporating intermittent fasting into your way of eating, your weekly meal plans will look different as well.

————

NOTE: Meal plans are based on a single serving size for each recipe.

Sunday

PROTEIN: 48 g
NET CARBS: 29 g
FATS: 178 g

Breakfast:
Asparagus Scramble

Keto Coffee (combine
1 cup hot coffee, ¼ cup
unsweetened almond
milk, 1 tablespoon hemp
protein powder, and
1 tablespoon refined
coconut oil in a blender;
cover and blend until
frothy and well combined).

Lunch:
Spinach Salad with
2 tablespoons toasted
walnuts

Snacks:
Tahini Dip: Combine
1½ tablespoons tahini,
2 teaspoons lemon juice,
1 tablespoon olive oil, a
dash of salt, and a dash of
garlic powder. Serve with
½ cup cucumber slices.

Dinner:
Grilled Cauliflower Steaks
with Romesco Sauce and
Toasted Nuts. Serve with
1 cup torn kale sautéed
in 2 tablespoons olive oil
until wilted; sprinkle with
1 teaspoon toasted
sesame seeds, 1
tablespoon hemp seeds,
and a dash of salt and
pepper.

Monday

PROTEIN: 59 g
NET CARBS: 27 g
FATS: 175 g

Breakfast:
*Matcha Latte with Yogurt
and Berries:* Mix one
5.3-ounce carton of nut
milk or coconut milk plain
unsweetened yogurt
with 1 tablespoon hemp
protein powder. Top with
¼ cup fresh blueberries,
¼ cup fresh raspberries,
2 tablespoons toasted
shredded coconut, and
1 tablespoon hemp seeds.

Lunch:
Tomato-Olive Salad:
Layer 1 cup fresh spinach,
½ cup grape tomatoes,
¼ cup chopped
cucumber, ¼ cup fresh
basil, ¼ cup chopped
kalamata olives,
2 tablespoons toasted
pine nuts, and
1 tablespoon thinly sliced
green onion tops. Whisk
2 tablespoons olive oil,
1 tablespoon tahini, and
1 tablespoon white wine
vinegar until smooth.
Drizzle over salad. Top
with 2 ounces canned
albacore tuna, drained
and flaked.

Snacks:
Coconut-Almond Balls

Dinner:
Grilled Romaine and
Avocado Caesar Salad
with Eggs

Tuesday

PROTEIN: 37 g
NET CARBS: 29 g
FATS: 185 g

Breakfast:
Greens Frittata with
¼ of an avocado

Lunch:
Antipasto Kabobs: Sauté
¾ cup each 1½-inch
pieces eggplant and
zucchini in 2 tablespoons
olive oil over medium
heat for 5 minutes. Set
aside until cool. Thread
vegetables onto skewers
with 6 cherry tomatoes
and 6 green olives. Whisk
3 tablespoons avocado
mayonnaise, 1 tablespoon
olive oil, and 1 teaspoon
Dijon-style mustard. Stir
in 2 tablespoons chopped
fresh basil and serve with
kabobs for dipping.

Snacks:
⅓ cup vegan chive
cream cheese–style
spread mixed with
1 tablespoon hemp
protein powder. Serve
with ½ cup cucumber
slices.

Dinner:
Pesto Zoodle Bowls

Wednesday PROTEIN: 72 g NET CARBS: 28 g FATS: 184 g	**Thursday** PROTEIN: 50 g NET CARBS: 28 g FATS: 178 g	**Friday** PROTEIN: 44 g NET CARBS: 25 g FATS: 185 g	**Saturday** PROTEIN: 39 g NET CARBS: 29 g FATS: 190 g

Wednesday

Breakfast:
Chia Pudding Breakfast Bowls

Lunch:
Cucumber, Radish, and Snap Pea Salad

Snacks:
Strawberry Protein Shake: Combine 1 cup fresh spinach, ¾ cup unsweetened almond milk, ¾ cup sliced fresh strawberries, ½ cup ice cubes, 2 tablespoons hemp protein powder, and 1 tablespoon flaxseed oil in a blender. Cover and blend until smooth. If desired, blend in a few drops of liquid stevia. Serve with ⅓ cup toasted walnuts.

Dinner:
Lemon-Garlic Salmon with Broccoli Rabe. Serve with spinach salad (1½ cups fresh spinach topped with 1 tablespoon toasted pine nuts and 2 teaspoons snipped fresh chives. Whisk together 2 tablespoons olive oil and 1 tablespoon lemon juice; drizzle over salad).

Thursday

Breakfast:
Veggie Fried Egg: In a small skillet, fry 2 eggs, sprinkled with salt and pepper, in 4 teaspoons ghee until desired doneness. Remove and keep warm. Sauté ¾ cup fresh baby spinach and 1 tablespoon thinly sliced green onion tops in 1 tablespoon olive oil for 30 seconds. Spoon over eggs. Serve with Keto Coffee (Combine 1 cup hot coffee, ¼ cup unsweetened almond milk, 1 tablespoon hemp protein powder, and 1 tablespoon refined coconut oil in a blender. Cover and blend until frothy.

Lunch:
Cucumber-Basil Lettuce Wraps: Stack 4 large Bibb lettuce leaves into 2 stacks of 2 leaves each. Divide ½ cup fresh basil, ½ cup thinly sliced cucumber, ¼ cup chopped red bell pepper, ¼ cup toasted pine nuts, and 2 tablespoons hemp seeds between lettuce stacks; sprinkle with black pepper. Spoon ¼ cup vegan chive cream cheese–style spread atop vegetables. Roll up.

Snacks:
2 servings Coconut-Almond Balls with 1 cup unsweetened almond milk

Dinner:
Roasted Beets and Greens (sprinkle with an additional 2 tablespoons chopped toasted walnuts) with 1 avocado

Friday

Breakfast:
Baked Cheesy Avocado: Halve and pit 1 avocado. Place, cut side up, on a foil-lined baking sheet; sprinkle with salt and pepper. Bake at 325°F for 8 to 10 minutes or until warm. Top with ½ cup Kite Hill jalapeño cream cheese–style spread; bake 1 minute more. Serve warm. Serve with 1 hard-cooked egg, peeled and sprinkled lightly with salt and pepper.

Lunch:
Ricotta-Kale Stuffed Tomato: Cut top off a large tomato. Scoop out most of the flesh and seeds and save for another use. Massage ⅔ cup torn kale with 2 tablespoons olive oil, 1 teaspoon lemon juice, and a dash of salt and pepper. Stir in ½ cup vegan ricotta-style cheese. Spoon into tomato; sprinkle with 1 tablespoon thinly sliced green onion tops. Serve with 6 large green olives.

Snacks:
½ cup roasted macadamia nuts

Dinner:
Smoked Trout Lettuce Wraps

Saturday

Breakfast:
Quick Egg-Chard Scramble with Matcha Latte

Lunch:
Tomato-Avocado Wraps: Spread 1 Sunfoods or Nuco brand coconut wrap with 2 tablespoons avocado mayonnaise mixed with ⅛ teaspoon chili powder. Top with 1 piece romaine lettuce, 2 small tomato slices, ½ avocado, sliced, and 2 tablespoons sliced black olives. Roll up.

Snacks:
Spiced Coconut Mixed Nuts

Dinner:
Stuffed Zucchini. Serve with spinach salad (1½ cups fresh spinach topped with 2 tablespoons hemp seeds, 1 tablespoon toasted pine nuts, and 2 teaspoons snipped fresh chives. Whisk together 2 tablespoons olive oil and 1 tablespoon lemon juice and drizzle over salad).

Sunday	Monday	Tuesday	
PROTEIN: 37 g NET CARBS: 53 g FATS: 191 g	PROTEIN: 61 g NET CARBS: 32 g FATS: 179 g	PROTEIN: 45 g NET CARBS: 49 g FATS: 176 g	

Sunday

Breakfast:
Berry-Cream Parfaits with Toasted Coconut Topping

Lunch:
Spring Veggie Lettuce Wraps. Serve with 2 ounces no-sugar-added smoked salmon

Snacks:
½ cup roasted macadamia nuts

Dinner:
Moroccan Vegetable Tagine with Olives and Cinnamon-Ghee Almonds

Monday

Breakfast:
Strawberry Cream Cheese Breakfast Wrap: Spread 1 Sunfoods or Nuco brand coconut wrap with 2 tablespoons plain vegan cream cheese–style spread (Kite Hill). Top with ½ cup arugula, ¼ cup chopped strawberries, and 3 tablespoons toasted sliced almonds. Roll up; cut crosswise into 1-inch slices. Serve with *Keto Coffee:* Combine 1 cup hot coffee, ¼ cup unsweetened almond milk, 1 tablespoon hemp protein powder, and 1 tablespoon refined coconut oil in a blender; cover and blend until frothy and well combined).

Lunch:
Warm German Brussels Sprout Salad. Serve with ⅓ cup roasted almonds.

Snacks:
Baked Avocado Fries with Smoky Tomato Mayo

Dinner:
Salmon Tacos

Tuesday

Breakfast:
Vegetable Hash with Fried Eggs

Lunch:
Cabbage-Fennel Salad: Toss 1 cup shredded cabbage with ½ cup thin strips fennel bulb, ¼ cup coarsely shredded carrot, 2 tablespoons chopped cilantro, 2 tablespoons avocado oil, 1 tablespoon cider vinegar, ⅛ teaspoon salt, and a pinch of black pepper. Stir in half of a chopped avocado.

Snacks:
Spirulina Super Smoothie

Dinner:
Butter Cauliflower. Serve with salad (1½ cups spinach topped with 4 cherry tomatoes, 2 tablespoons hemp seeds, and 1 tablespoon thinly sliced green onion tops. Whisk together 2 tablespoons olive oil and 1 tablespoon lemon juice. Drizzle over salad).

Wednesday	Thursday	Friday	Saturday
PROTEIN: 42 g NET CARBS: 51 g FATS: 175 g	PROTEIN: 47 g NET CARBS: 52 g FATS: 196 g	PROTEIN: 98 g NET CARBS: 40 g FATS: 154 g	PROTEIN: 53 g NET CARBS: 47 g FATS: 184 g

Wednesday

Breakfast:
Cucumber "Toast" Bites with Avocado and Coconut (AIP). Serve with Matcha Latte.

Lunch:
Nut and Veggie Bento Box: ½ cup mixed toasted pistachio nuts, macadamia nuts, and almonds; ¼ cup soft truffle dill and chive vegan cheese; ¾ cup sliced cucumbers, bell pepper strips, and/or cherry tomatoes to dip in cheese; ½ cup raspberries; 6 green olives

Snacks:
Coconut-Raspberry Smoothie

Dinner:
Italian Egg-Stuffed Portobello Mushrooms. Serve with Roasted Broccoli with Lemon and Olives.

Thursday

Breakfast:
Baked Cheesy Avocado: Place 1 halved and pitted avocado, cut side up, on a foil-lined baking sheet; sprinkle with salt and pepper. Bake at 325°F for 8 to 10 minutes or until warm. Top with ½ cup Kite Hill jalapeño cream cheese–style spread; bake 1 minute more. Serve warm.

Lunch:
Cauliflower Hummus Wraps. Serve with ½ cup walnuts.

Snacks:
Two hard-cooked eggs; peel and cut eggs in half. Scoop yolks into a small bowl; add 2 tablespoons avocado mayonnaise and a pinch of black pepper. Mash with a fork. Spoon back into egg whites.

Dinner:
Thai Vegetable Cashew Curry with Coconut

Friday

Breakfast:
Keto Cereal: Combine ½ cup mixed chopped toasted unsalted macadamia nuts, chopped roasted salted pistachio nuts, and chopped toasted pecans with 2 tablespoons toasted shredded coconut. Add 1 tablespoon hemp seeds and 1 teaspoon finely shredded orange peel. Serve in a bowl with ¼ cup chopped fresh strawberries and ⅓ cup unsweetened coconut or almond milk.

Lunch:
Albacore Tuna Salad with Grapefruit and Avocado

Snacks:
Strawberry Protein Shake: Combine 1 cup fresh spinach, ¾ cup unsweetened almond milk, ¾ cup sliced fresh strawberries, ½ cup ice cubes, 2 tablespoons hemp protein powder, and 2 tablespoons flaxseed oil in a blender; cover and blend until smooth. If desired, blend in a few drops of liquid stevia.

Dinner:
Spicy Frittata Pizza with Spinach and Olives

Saturday

Breakfast:
Omelet with sautéed mushrooms, chard, and nut cheese

Lunch:
Tomato-Avocado Wraps: Spread 1 Sunfoods or Nuco brand coconut wrap with 2 tablespoons avocado mayonnaise mixed with ⅛ teaspoon chili powder. Top with 1 piece romaine lettuce, 2 small tomato slices, ½ avocado, sliced, and 2 tablespoons sliced black olives. Roll up.

Snacks:
⅓ cup roasted almonds; ⅓ cup fresh blueberries

Dinner:
Mushroom–Red Wine Ragout with Brussels Sprouts, Olives, and Herbs. Serve with salad (1½ cups spinach topped with 4 cherry tomatoes, 2 tablespoons hemp seeds, and 1 tablespoon thinly sliced green onion tops; whisk together 2 tablespoons olive oil and 1 tablespoon lemon juice. Drizzle over salad).

Sunday	Monday	Tuesday	
PROTEIN: 40 g NET CARBS: 52 g FATS: 167 g	PROTEIN: 58 g NET CARBS: 40 g FATS: 178 g	PROTEIN: 45 g NET CARBS: 49 g FATS: 176 g	

week 3

Sunday

Breakfast:
Vegetable Hash with Fried Eggs

Lunch:
Coconut Mushroom Simmer

Snacks:
Tahini Dip: Combine 1 tablespoon tahini, 2 teaspoons lemon juice, 1 teaspoon olive oil, a dash of salt, and a dash of garlic powder. Serve with ¾ cup bell pepper strips.

Dinner:
Roasted Eggplant with Beet-Tahini Yogurt and Toasted Pumpkin Seeds. Serve with kale salad (massage 1½ cups torn fresh kale with 2 tablespoons sesame oil and ⅛ teaspoon coarse salt until kale is wilted. Toss with 1 tablespoon white wine vinegar. Top with ¼ cup chopped cucumber and 2 tablespoons toasted pine nuts).

Monday

Breakfast:
Yogurt and Berries: Mix one 5.3-ounce carton nut milk or coconut milk plain unsweetened yogurt with 1 tablespoon hemp protein powder. Top with ¼ cup fresh blueberries, ¼ cup fresh raspberries, 2 tablespoons toasted shredded coconut, and 1 tablespoon hemp seeds. Serve with *Keto Coffee:* Combine 1 cup hot coffee, ¼ cup unsweetened almond milk, 1 tablespoon hemp protein powder, and 1 tablespoon refined coconut oil in a blender; cover and blend until frothy and well combined.

Lunch:
Raspberry Super Salad with Toasted Coconut. Serve with ½ cup toasted walnuts.

Snacks:
Guacamole and Veggies: Mash ½ ripe avocado with 1 tablespoon avocado oil, 2 teaspoons spirulina powder, 1 tablespoon lime juice, ⅛ teaspoon coarse salt, and ½ minced garlic clove. Serve with 10 cherry tomatoes.

Dinner:
Cauliflower Fried Rice Bowls

Tuesday

Breakfast:
Asparagus Scramble. Serve with Spirulina Super Smoothie.

Lunch:
Sardine-Stuffed Tomatoes

Snacks:
Spiced Coconut Mixed Nuts

Dinner:
Zucchini and Mushroom Satay. Serve with Creamed Kale.

Wednesday	Thursday	Friday	Saturday
PROTEIN: 52 g NET CARBS: 47 g FATS: 165 g	PROTEIN: 68 g NET CARBS: 44 g FATS: 166 g	PROTEIN: 47 g NET CARBS: 50 g FATS: 175 g	PROTEIN: 51 g NET CARBS: 38 g FATS: 182 g

Wednesday

Breakfast:
Baked Salsa Avocado: Place half of a pitted avocado on a foil-lined baking sheet; sprinkle with salt and pepper. Bake at 325°F for 8 to 10 minutes or until warm. Top with ¼ cup Kite Hill jalapeño cream cheese–style spread; bake 1 minute more. Top with 2 tablespoons fresh salsa; serve warm. Serve with Matcha Latte.

Lunch:
Niçoise Salad Wraps: Layer 4 bibb lettuce leaves to make two stacks of two leaves. Divide ½ cup steamed green beans, ¼ cup halved grape tomatoes, 2 ounces canned white tuna in oil (drained and flaked), 1 sliced hard-cooked egg, 2 tablespoons chopped Niçoise or kalamata olives, and 1 tablespoon chopped shallot between leaf stacks. Whisk together 2 tablespoons olive oil, 1 tablespoon lemon juice, and ½ teaspoon Dijon-style mustard; drizzle over filling.

Snacks:
Coconut-Raspberry Smoothie

Dinner:
Sheet-Pan Veggies with Nut-Free Olive-Basil Pesto (AIP). Serve with Kale Chips with Toasted Sesame Seeds, Rice Vinegar, Lime Juice, and Sesame Oil.

Thursday

Breakfast:
Baked Cheesy Avocado: Place 1 halved and pitted avocado, cut side up, on a foil-lined baking sheet; sprinkle with salt and pepper. Bake at 325°F for 8 to 10 minutes or until warm. Top with ½ cup Kite Hill jalapeño cream cheese–style spread; bake 1 minute more. Serve warm.

Lunch:
Roasted Beet-Cheese-Basil Caprese with Avocado and Toasted Almonds

Snacks:
Strawberry-Avocado Smoothies (add 2 tablespoons hemp protein powder to recipe before blending). Serve with 2 tablespoons macadamia nuts.

Dinner:
Catfish Po'Boy Wraps with Celery Root Slaw

Friday

Breakfast:
Veggie Fried Egg: In a small skillet, fry 1 egg, sprinkled with salt and pepper, in 2 teaspoons ghee until yolk is to desired doneness. Remove from skillet; keep warm. Sauté ½ cup bite-size bell pepper strips in 1 tablespoon olive oil for 3 minutes. Remove from the heat; stir in ¾ cup fresh baby spinach and 1 tablespoon thinly sliced green onion tops. Spoon over egg.

Lunch:
Egg Salad–Stuffed Avocado: Remove 1 tablespoon flesh from half of a pitted avocado; mash and mix with 1 tablespoon avocado mayonnaise. Stir in 1 chopped hard-cooked egg, ½ cup chopped fresh spinach, 2 tablespoons chopped red bell pepper, and 1 tablespoon sliced green onion tops. Stuff into the avocado half. Sprinkle with salt and pepper.

Snacks:
Coconut-Raspberry Smoothie (sprinkle the serving with 1 tablespoon hemp seeds). Serve with ¼ cup roasted almonds.

Dinner:
Meatless Mexican Kale Enchiladas

Saturday

Breakfast:
Roasted Beet with Avocado, Grapefruit, and Pickled Red Onion. Serve with ¼ cup toasted pecans.

Lunch:
Avocado-Kale Salad: Massage 2 cups torn kale with 3 tablespoons olive oil, ¼ teaspoon coarse salt, and ⅛ teaspoon black pepper until wilted. Toss with 1 tablespoon lime juice. Top with ½ sliced avocado, ¼ cup red bell pepper strips, 2 ounces flaked sugar-free smoked salmon, and 2 tablespoons hemp seeds.

Snacks:
Two hard-cooked eggs; peel and cut eggs in half. Scoop yolks into a small bowl; add 2 tablespoons avocado mayonnaise and a pinch of black pepper. Mash with a fork. Spoon back into egg whites.

Dinner:
Individual Cauliflower Plank Pizzas

Sunday	Monday	Tuesday	
PROTEIN: 64 g NET CARBS: 40 g FATS: 175 g	PROTEIN: 69 g NET CARBS: 44 g FATS: 161 g	PROTEIN: 43 g NET CARBS: 52 g FATS: 174 g	

Sunday

Breakfast:
Quick Egg-Chard Scramble. Serve with *Strawberry Protein Shake:* Combine 1 cup fresh spinach, ¾ cup unsweetened almond milk, ¾ cup sliced fresh strawberries, ½ cup ice cubes, 2 tablespoons hemp protein powder, and 2 tablespoons flaxseed oil in a blender; cover and blend until smooth. If desired, blend in a few drops of liquid stevia.

Lunch:
Crispy Brussels Sprouts with Fish Sauce and Lime

Snacks:
Baked Avocado Fries with Smoky Tomato Mayo

Dinner:
Grilled Halibut with Grapefruit Salsa. Serve with Tangy Green Beans with Olives.

Monday

Breakfast:
Lox and Egg Scramble with Dilled Almond-Milk Yogurt. Serve with Matcha Latte.

Lunch:
Asian Cabbage-Mushroom Soup. Serve with ⅓ cup walnuts.

Snacks:
½ cup cucumber slices; ⅓ cup chive vegan cream cheese–style spread mixed with 1 tablespoon hemp protein powder. Spread on cucumber.

Dinner:
Coconut Veggie Stir-Fry with Cauliflower Rice

Tuesday

Breakfast:
Berry-Cream Parfaits with Toasted Coconut Topping

Lunch:
Cucumber-Basil Wraps: Spread 1 Sunfoods or Nuco brand coconut wrap with 2 tablespoons vegan chive cream cheese–style spread. Top with ¼ cup fresh spinach, ¼ cup fresh basil, ¼ cup thinly sliced cucumber, 2 tablespoons chopped red bell pepper, 2 tablespoons toasted pine nuts, and 1 tablespoon hemp seeds; sprinkle with black pepper. Roll up.

Snacks:
⅓ cup roasted almonds; ¼ cup fresh blueberries

Dinner:
Poached Eggs over Tomato-Olive-Caper Sauce with Fresh Oregano. Serve with salad (1 cup spinach, ½ cup arugula, 2 tablespoons chopped bell pepper, 2 tablespoons toasted chopped walnuts. Whisk together 2 tablespoons olive oil and 1 tablespoon white wine vinegar; drizzle over salad).

Wednesday	Thursday	Friday	Saturday
PROTEIN: 47 g NET CARBS: 45 g FATS: 180 g	PROTEIN: 61 g NET CARBS: 39 g FATS: 172 g	PROTEIN: 59 g NET CARBS: 49 g FATS: 164 g	PROTEIN: 41 g NET CARBS: 51 g FATS: 176 g

Wednesday

Breakfast:
Egg-o-cado

Lunch:
Wilted Cabbage and Beet Chip Buddha Bowls. Sprinkle with 2 tablespoons hemp seeds.

Snacks:
Two hard-cooked eggs; peel and cut eggs in half. Scoop yolks into a small bowl; add 2 tablespoons avocado mayonnaise and a pinch of black pepper. Mash with a fork. Spoon back into egg whites.

Dinner:
Spaghetti Squash with Pine Nuts and Basil. Serve with salad (combine ½ cup thinly sliced cucumber and 1 tablespoon thin slivers red onion. Whisk together 2 tablespoons nut milk or coconut milk plain unsweetened yogurt, 2 teaspoons olive oil, 2 teaspoons white wine vinegar, and ⅛ teaspoon coarse salt; stir into cucumber mixture).

Thursday

Breakfast:
Keto Cereal: Combine ½ cup mixed chopped toasted unsalted macadamia nuts, chopped roasted salted pistachio nuts, and chopped toasted pecans with 2 tablespoons toasted shredded coconut. Add 1 tablespoon hemp seeds and 1 teaspoon finely shredded orange peel. Serve in a bowl with ¼ cup chopped fresh strawberries and ⅓ cup unsweetened coconut or almond milk. Serve with *Keto Coffee.* (See Week 1, Thursday.)

Lunch:
Smoked Trout Lettuce Wraps

Snacks:
Green Protein Smoothie: In a blender combine ¾ cup unsweetened almond milk; ¾ cup torn, trimmed fresh Swiss chard leaves or spinach; ½ cup grapefruit sections, ½ cup ice cubes, and 2 tablespoons hemp protein powder. Cover and blend until smooth.

Dinner:
Chinese Fried Cabbage-and-Egg-Stuffed Peppers. Serve with salad (1 cup spinach, ½ cup arugula, 2 tablespoons chopped bell pepper, 2 tablespoons toasted chopped walnuts. Whisk together 2 tablespoons olive oil and 1 tablespoon white wine vinegar; drizzle over salad).

Friday

Breakfast:
Greens Frittata. Serve with Strawberry-Avocado Smoothies.

Lunch:
Sesame-Lemon Fennel-Cucumber Slaw. Serve with 3 ounces canned albacore tuna, drained and flaked.

Snacks:
Tahini Dip: Mix 2 tablespoons tahini, 2 teaspoons lemon juice, 1 tablespoon olive oil, a pinch of salt, and a pinch of garlic powder. Serve with ¾ cup bell pepper strips.

Dinner:
Roasted Cauliflower Tacos

Saturday

Breakfast:
Strawberry Cream Cheese Breakfast Wrap: Spread 1 Sunfoods or Nuco brand coconut wrap with 2 tablespoons plain vegan cream cheese–style spread (Kite Hill). Top with ½ cup arugula, ¼ cup chopped strawberries, 3 tablespoons toasted sliced almonds, and 1 tablespoon hemp seeds. Roll up; cut crosswise into 1-inch slices.

Lunch:
Italian Cauliflower Rice Soup. Serve with Kale Chips with Toasted Sesame Seeds, Rice Vinegar, Lime, and Sesame Oil

Snacks:
⅓ cup roasted macadamia nuts; ¼ cup fresh raspberries

Dinner:
Grilled Romaine and Avocado Caesar Salad with Eggs

acknowledgments

Amber, Solomon, and Shiloh, thank you for being my core and my heart. "I love you" and "thank you" do not encapsulate my feelings toward you and all that you deserve. With every breath and beyond, I am yours.

My team: Andrea, Ashley, Yvette, and Emily. You are part of my family and my closest friends. Thank you for your tireless devotion and passion for the patients we care so much about.

My patients: Thank you for letting me be a part of your sacred journey into wellness. I do not take that responsibility lightly. Serving you is an honor.

Heather, Megan, Marian, and everyone at Avery and Waterbury: You are the best team I could have dreamed of. Thank you so much for believing in me and making this book come to fruition.

Jason, Colleen, and my mindbodygreen family: Thank you for all you have done for me. For giving me a voice and a home. I am eternally grateful.

Dr. Terry Wahls, Dr. Alejandro Junger, Dr. Josh Axe, and Dr. Frank Lipman: Thank you for being my heroes, mentors, and friends in this space of wellness and food.

Melissa Hartwig: This book wouldn't be as great as it is, if it weren't for you. Thank you for your friendship and guidance.

Lee, Jason, Ed, and my Amplify family: Thank you for being my teachers, friends, and core community.

Finally, thank you to everyone in the functional-medicine and wellness world. Many of you are so special to me. Together we are changing the world for the better. You are seen and appreciated immensely.

notes

Introduction: The Ketotarian Manifesto

1   National Institute of Mental Health, "Mental Illness," https://www.nimh.nih.gov/health/statistics/prevalence/any-mental-illness-ami-among-us-adults.shtml.

2   C. Pritchard et al., "Changing Patterns of Neurological Mortality in the 10 Major Developed Countries—1979-2010," *Public Health* 126, no. 4 (April 2013): 357-368; doi: 10.1016/j.puhe.2012.12.018, https://www.ncbi.nlm.nih.gov/pubmed/23601790.

3   CDC, "*QuickStats:* Suicide Rates for Teens Aged 15-19 Years, by Sex—United States, 1975-2015," *MMWR Weekly* 66, no. 30 (August 4, 2017): 816, https://www.cdc.gov/mmwr/volumes/66/wr/mm6630a6.htm.

4   D. Munro, "U.S. Healthcare Ranked Dead Last Compared to 10 Other Countries," *Forbes,* June 16, 2014, https://www.forbes.com/sites/danmunro/2014/06/16/u-s-healthcare-ranked-dead-last-compared-to-10-other-countries/#1591ceb3576f.

5   B. Starfield, "Is US Health Really the Best in the World?," *JAMA* 284, no. 4 (July 6, 2000): 483-485, doi:10.1001/jama.284.4.483, https://jamanetwork.com/journals/jama/article-abstract/192908.

6   America's Health Rankings, *Annual Report 2017,* https://assets.americashealthrankings.org/app/uploads/2017annualreport.pdf.

7   L. Girion et al., "Drug Deaths Now Outnumber Traffic Fatalities in U.S., Data Show," *Los Angeles Times,* September 17, 2011, http://articles.latimes.com/2011/sep/17/local/la-me-drugs-epidemic-20110918.

8   B. Starfield, "Is US Health Really the Best in the World," *JAMA* 284, no. 4 (2000): 483-485.

9   J. Lazarou et al., "Incidence of Adverse Drug Reactions in Hospitalized Patients: A Meta-Analysis of Prospective Studies," *JAMA* 279, no. 15 (April 15, 1998): 1200-1205, https://www.ncbi.nlm.nih.gov/pubmed/9555760.

10 K. Adams et al., "Nutrition Education in U.S. Medical Schools: Latest Update of a National Survey," *Academic Medicine* 85, no. 9 (September 2010): 1537-1542, https://www.aamc.org/download/451374/data/nutriritoneducationinusmedschools.pdf.

11 K. Adams et al., "The State of Nutrition Education at US Medical Schools," *Journal of Biomedical Education* 2015 (2015), Article ID 357627, 7 pages, http://dx.doi.org/10.1155/2015/357627, https://www.hindawi.com/journals/jbe/2015/357627/.

12 M. Castillo et al., "Basic Nutrition Knowledge of Recent Medical Graduates Entering a Pediatric Residency Program," *International Journal of Adolescent Medicine and Health* 28, no. 4 (November 1, 2016): 357-361, doi: 10.1515/ijamh-2015-0019, https://www.ncbi.nlm.nih.gov/pubmed/26234947.

Chapter 1: The Ketogenic Diet (for Better and Worse)

1   J. Medina and A. Tabernero, "Lactate Utilization by Brain Cells and Its Role in CNS Development," *Journal of Neuroscience Research* 79 (2005): 2-10, https://www.researchgate.net/publication/234095885.

2   S. Schilling et al., "Plasma Lipids and Cerebral Small Vessel Disease," *Neurology* 83, no. 20 (November 11, 2014): 1844-1852, doi: 10.1212/WNL.0000000000000980, https://www.ncbi

.nlm.nih.gov/pubmed/25320101; I. Schatz et al., "Cholesterol and All-Cause Mortality in Elderly People from the Honolulu Heart Program: A Cohort Study," *Lancet* 358, no. 9279 (August 4, 2001): 351–355, http://www.thelancet.com/journals/lancet /article/PIIS0140673601055532/abstract.

3   C. Ramsden et al., "Re-evaluation of the Traditional Diet-Heart Hypothesis: Analysis of Recovered Data from Minnesota Coronary Experiment (1968–73)," *British Medical Journal* (April 12, 2016): 353, doi: https://doi.org/10.1136/bmj.i1246, http://www.bmj .com/content/353/bmj.i1246.

4   A. Feranil et al., "Coconut Oil Predicts a Beneficial Lipid Profile in Pre-Menopausal Women in the Philippines," *Asia Pacific Journal of Clinical Nutrition* 20, no. 2 (2011): 190–195, https://www.ncbi .nlm.nih.gov/pmc/articles/PMC3146349/.

5   C. Cox et al., "Effects of Dietary Coconut Oil, Butter and Safflower Oil on Plasma Lipids, Lipoproteins and Lathosterol Levels," *European Journal of Clinical Nutrition* 52, no. 9 (September 1998): 650–654, https://www.ncbi.nlm.nih.gov/pubmed/9756121.

6   R. de Souza et al., "Intake of Saturated and Trans Unsaturated Fatty Acids and Risk of All Cause Mortality, Cardiovascular Disease, and Type 2 Diabetes: Systematic Review and Meta-Analysis of Observational Studies," *British Medical Journal* (August 12, 2015): 351, doi: https://doi.org/10.1136/bmj.h3978, http://www.bmj.com/content/351/bmj.h3978.

7   V. Veum et al., "Visceral Adiposity and Metabolic Syndrome after Very High-Fat and Low-Fat Isocaloric Diets: A Randomized Controlled Trial," *American Journal of Clinical Nutrition* 105, no. 1 (January 1, 2017): 85–89, doi: 10.3945 /ajcn.115.123463, http://ajcn.nutrition.org/content /early/2016/11/30/ajcn.115.123463.abstract.

8   University of North Carolina Health Care, "Did Butter Get a Bad Rap?," April 12, 2016, https:// www.eurekalert.org/pub_releases/2016-04 /uonc-dbg041216.php.

9   J. Medina and A. Tabernero, "Lactate Utilization by Brain Cells and Its Role in CNS Development."

10   K. Nylen et al., "The Effects of a Ketogenic Diet on ATP Concentrations and the Number of Hippocampal Mitochondria in Aldh5a1(-/-) Mice," *Biochimica et Biophysica Acta* 1790, no. 3 (March 2009): 208–212, doi: 10.1016/j.bbagen.2008.12.005, https://www.ncbi.nlm.nih.gov/pubmed/19168117.

11   Z. Zhao, "A Ketogenic Diet as a Potential Novel Therapeutic Intervention in Amyotrophic Lateral Sclerosis," *BMC Neuroscience* 7 (April 3, 2006): 29, https://www.ncbi.nlm.nih.gov/pmc/articles /PMC1488864/.

12   "Autoimmune Disease Statistics," https:// www.aarda.org/news-information/statistics/.

13   "Adrenal Insufficiency & Addison's Disease," https://www.niddk.nih.gov/health-information /endocrine-diseases/adrenal-insufficiency -addisons-disease.

14   J. Milder et al., "Acute Oxidative Stress and Systemic Nrf2 Activation by the Ketogenic Diet," *Neurobiology of Disease* 40, no. 1 (October 2010): 238–244, doi: 10.1016/j.nbd.2010.05.030, https:// www.ncbi.nlm.nih.gov/pubmed/20594978.

15   T.-D. Kannaganti, "Inflammatory Bowel Disease and the NLRP3 Inflammasome," *New England Journal of Medicine* 377 (August 17, 2017): 694–696, doi: 10.1056/NEJMcibr170653, http://www.nejm.org /doi/full/10.1056/NEJMcibr1706536.

16   H. Bae et al., "ß-Hydroxybutyrate Suppresses Inflammasome Formation by Ameliorating Endoplasmic Reticulum Stress via AMPK Activation," *Oncotarget* 7, no. 41 (October 11, 2016): 66444–66454, https://www.ncbi.nlm.nih.gov/pmc/articles /PMC5341812/; A. Salminen et al., "AMP-Activated Protein Kinase Inhibits NF-B Signaling and Inflammation: Impact on Healthspan and Lifespan," *Journal of Molecular Medicine* 89, no. 7 (July 2011): 667–676, https://www.ncbi.nlm.nih.gov/pmc /articles/PMC3111671/.

17   S.-P. Fu et al., "Anti-Inflammatory Effects of BHBA in Both In Vivo and In Vitro Parkinson's Disease Models Are Mediated by GPR109A-Dependent Mechanisms," *Journal of Neuroinflammation* 12, no. 9 (2015), https://jneuroinflammation.biomedcentral .com/articles/10.1186/s12974-014-0230-3.

18   M. McCarty et al., "Ketosis May Promote Brain Macroautophagy by Activating Sirt1 and Hypoxia-Inducible Factor-1," *Medical Hypotheses* 85, no. 5 (November 2015): 631–639, doi: 10.1016 /j.mehy.2015.08.002, https://www.ncbi.nlm.nih.gov /pubmed/26306884.

19   I. Björkhem and S. Meaney, "Brain Cholesterol: Long Secret Life behind a Barrier," *Arteriosclerosis, Thrombosis, and Vascular Biology* 24 (2004): 806–815, http://atvb.ahajournals.org/content /24/5/806.full.

20   C. Chang et al., "Essential Fatty Acids and Human Brain," *Acta Neurologica Taiwanica* 18, no. 4 (December 2009): 231–241, https://www.ncbi.nlm .nih.gov/pubmed/20329590.

21   Iowa State University, "Cholesterol-Reducing Drugs May Lessen Brain Function, Says ISU Researcher," February 23, 2009, http://www.public.iastate .edu/~nscentral/news/2009/feb/shin.shtml.

22   A. Hadhazy, "Think Twice: How the Gut's 'Second

Brain' Influences Mood and Well-Being," *Scientific American*, February 12, 2010, https://www.scientificamerican.com/article/gut-second-brain/.

23 V. Perry, "Contribution of Systemic Inflammation to Chronic Neurodegeneration," *Acta Neuropathologica* 120, no. 3 (September 2010): 277–286, doi: 10.1007/s00401-010-0722-x, https://www.ncbi.nlm.nih.gov/pubmed/20644946.

24 M. Block and J. Hong, "Microglia and Inflammation-Mediated Neurodegeneration: Multiple Triggers with a Common Mechanism," *Progress in Neurobiology* 76, no. 2 (June 2005): 77–98, https://www.ncbi.nlm.nih.gov/pubmed/16081203.

25 O. Schiepers et al., "Cytokines and Major Depression," *Progress in Neuro-psychopharmacology and Biological Psychiatry* 29, no. 2 (February 2005): 201–217, https://www.ncbi.nlm.nih.gov/pubmed/15694227.

26 O. Abdel-Salam et al., "Oxidative Stress in a Model of Toxic Demyelination in Rat Brain: The Effect of Piracetam and Vinpocetine," *Neurochemical Research* 36, no. 6 (June 2011): 1062–1072, https://doi.org/10.1007/s11064-011-0450-1, https://link.springer.com/article/10.1007%2Fs11064-011-0450-1?wt_mc=Affiliate.CommissionJunction.3.EPR1089.DeepLink&utm_medium=affiliate&utm_source=commission_junction&utm_campaign=3_nsn6445_deeplink&utm_content=deeplink#citeas.

27 G. Ede, "Ketogenic Diets for Psychiatric Disorders: A New 2017 Review," *Psychology Today*, June 30, 2017, https://www.psychologytoday.com/blog/diagnosis-diet/201706/ketogenic-diets-psychiatric-disorders-new-2017-review.

28 A. Swidsinski et al., "Reduced Mass and Diversity of the Colonic Microbiome in Patients with Multiple Sclerosis and Their Improvement with Ketogenic Diet." *Front Microbiol*, 2017:8:1141. Published 2017 Jun 28. doi: 10.3389/fmicb.2017.01141.ncbi.nlm.nih.gov/pmc/articles/PMC5488402/

29 S. Thaler et al., "Neuroprotection by Acetoacetate and -Hydroxybutyrate against NMDA-Induced RGC Damage in Rat—Possible Involvement of Kynurenic Acid," *Graefe's Archive for Clinical and Experimental Ophthalmology* 248, no. 12 (December 2010): 1729–1735, https://www.ncbi.nlm.nih.gov/pmc/articles/PMC2974203/.

30 M. Reger et al., "Effects of Beta-Hydroxybutyrate on Cognition in Memory-Impaired Adults," *Neurobiology of Aging* 25, no. 3 (March 2004): 311–314, https://www.ncbi.nlm.nih.gov/pubmed/15123336.

31 K. Tieu et al., "D-ß-Hydroxybutyrate Rescues Mitochondrial Respiration and Mitigates Features of Parkinson Disease," *Journal of Clinical Investigation* 112, no. 6 (September 15, 2003): 892–901, https://www.ncbi.nlm.nih.gov/pmc/articles/PMC193668/.

32 M. Morris et al., "Consumption of Fish and n-3 Fatty Acids and Risk of Incident Alzheimer Disease," *Archives of Neurology* 60, no. 7 (July 2003): 940–946, https://www.ncbi.nlm.nih.gov/pubmed/12873849.

33 T. Vanitallie et al., "Treatment of Parkinson Disease with Diet-Induced Hyperketonemia: A Feasibility Study," *Neurology* 64, no. 4 (February 2005): 728–730, https://www.ncbi.nlm.nih.gov/pubmed/15728303/.

34 A. Evangeliou et al., "Application of a Ketogenic Diet in Children with Autistic Behavior: Pilot Study," *Journal of Child Neurology* 18, no. 2 (February 2003): 113–118, https://www.ncbi.nlm.nih.gov/pubmed/12693778.

35 S. Henderson, "High Carbohydrate Diets and Alzheimer's Disease," *Medical Hypotheses* 62, no. 5 (2004): 689–700, https://www.ncbi.nlm.nih.gov/pubmed/15082091.

36 M. Prins, "Diet, Ketones and Neurotrauma," *Epilepsia* 49, suppl. 8 (November 2008): 111–113, https://www.ncbi.nlm.nih.gov/pmc/articles/PMC2652873/.

37 S. Masino and J. Rho, "Mechanisms of Ketogenic Diet Action," in J. Noebels et al., eds., *Jasper's Basic Mechanisms of the Epilepsies*, 4th ed. (Bethesda, MD: National Center for Biotechnology Information, 2012), https://www.ncbi.nlm.nih.gov/pubmed/22787591.

38 A. Bergqvist et al., "Fasting versus Gradual Initiation of the Ketogenic Diet: A Prospective, Randomized Clinical Trial of Efficacy," *Epilepsia* 46, no. 11 (November 2005): 1810–1819, https://www.ncbi.nlm.nih.gov/pubmed/16302862.

39 S. Kinsman et al., "Efficacy of the Ketogenic Diet for Intractable Seizure Disorders: Review of 58 Cases," *Epilepsia* 33, no. 6 (November–December 1992): 1132–1136, https://www.ncbi.nlm.nih.gov/pubmed/1464275/.

40 P. Azevedo de Lima et al., "Neurobiochemical Mechanisms of a Ketogenic Diet in Refractory Epilepsy," *Clinics (São Paulo)* 69, no. 10 (October 2014): 699–705, https://www.ncbi.nlm.nih.gov/pmc/articles/PMC4221309/.

41 A. McKenzie et al., "A Novel Intervention Including Individualized Nutritional Recommendations Reduces Hemoglobin A1c Level, Medication Use, and Weight in Type 2 Diabetes," *JMIR Diabetes* 2, no. 1 (January–June 2017):ie5, http://diabetes.jmir.org/2017/1/e5/.

42 C. Burns, "Higher Serum Glucose Levels Are Asso-

ciated with Cerebral Hypometabolism in Alzheimer Regions," *Neurology* 80, no. 17 (April 23, 2013): 1557–1564, doi: 10.1212/WNL.0b013e31828f17de, https://www.ncbi.nlm.nih.gov/pubmed/23535495.

43 A. Paoli, "Ketogenic Diet for Obesity: Friend or Foe?," *International Journal of Environmental Research and Public Health* 11, no. 2 (February 2014): 2092–2107, https://www.ncbi.nlm.nih.gov/pmc/articles/PMC3945587/.

44 https://jamanetwork.com/journals/jama/article-abstract/2669724?redirect=true.

45 F. McClernon, "The Effects of a Low-Carbohydrate Ketogenic Diet and a Low-Fat Diet on Mood, Hunger, and Other Self-Reported Symptoms," *Obesity (Silver Spring)* 15, no. 1 (January 2007): 182–187, https://www.ncbi.nlm.nih.gov/pubmed/17228046.

46 M. Hussein et al., "Long-Term Effects of a Ketogenic Diet in Obese Patients," *Experimental and Clinical Cardiology* 9, no. 3 (Fall 2004): 200–205, https://www.ncbi.nlm.nih.gov/pmc/articles/PMC2716748/.

47 N. Al-Zaid et al., "Low Carbohydrate Ketogenic Diet Enhances Cardiac Tolerance to Global Ischaemia," *Acta Cardiologica* 62, no. 4 (August 2007): 381–389, https://www.ncbi.nlm.nih.gov/pubmed/17824299.

48 "Cancer Facts & Figures 2017," https://www.cancer.org/research/cancer-facts-statistics/all-cancer-facts-figures/cancer-facts-figures-2017.html.

49 "Cancer Facts & Figures 2017"; E. Woolf et al., "Tumor Metabolism, the Ketogenic Diet and ß-Hydroxybutyrate: Novel Approaches to Adjuvant Brain Tumor Therapy," *Frontiers in Molecular Neuroscience* 9 (November 16, 2012): 122, https://www.ncbi.nlm.nih.gov/pubmed/27899882.

50 C. Otto et al., "Growth of Human Gastric Cancer Cells in Nude Mice Is Delayed by a Ketogenic Diet Supplemented with Omega-3 Fatty Acids and Medium-Chain Triglycerides," *BMC Cancer* 8 (April 30, 2008): 122, doi: 10.1186/1471-2407-8-122, https://www.ncbi.nlm.nih.gov/pubmed/18447912.

51 B. Allen et al., "Ketogenic Diets Enhance Oxidative Stress and Radio-Chemo-Therapy Responses in Lung Cancer Xenograft," *Clinical Cancer Research* 19, no. 14 (July 2013): 3905–3913, doi: 10.1158/1078-0432.CCR-12-0287, https://www.ncbi.nlm.nih.gov/pubmed/23743570.

52 S. Freedland et al., "Carbohydrate Restriction, Prostate Cancer Growth, and the Insulin-Like Growth Factor Axis," *Prostate* 68, no. 1 (January 1, 2008): 11–19, https://www.ncbi.nlm.nih.gov/pubmed/17999389.

53 J. March et al., "Drug/Diet Synergy for Managing Malignant Astrocytoma in Mice: 2-Deoxy-D-Glucose and the Restricted Ketogenic Diet," *Nutrition and Metabolism (London)* 5 (2008): 33, https://www.ncbi.nlm.nih.gov/pmc/articles/PMC2607273/.

54 J. Maroon et al., "The Role of Metabolic Therapy in Treating Glioblastoma Multiforme," *Surgical Neurology International* 6 (2015): 61, https://www.ncbi.nlm.nih.gov/pmc/articles/PMC4405891/.

55 W. Li et al., "Targeting AMPK for Cancer Prevention and Treatment," *Oncotarget* 6, no. 10 (April 10, 2015): 7365–7378, https://www.ncbi.nlm.nih.gov/pmc/articles/PMC4480686/.

56 E. Carmina, "PCOS: Metabolic Impact and Long-Term Management," *Minerva Ginecologica* 64, no. 6 (December 2012): 501–505, https://www.ncbi.nlm.nih.gov/pubmed/23232534.

57 G. Muscogiuri et al., "Current Insights into Inositol Isoforms, Mediterranean and Ketogenic Diets for Polycystic Ovary Syndrome: From Bench to Bedside," *Current Pharmaceutical Design* 22, no. 36 (2016): 5554–5557, https://www.ncbi.nlm.nih.gov/pubmed/27510483.

58 "Food Allergies: Reducing the Risks," https://www.fda.gov/ForConsumers/ConsumerUpdates/ucm089307.htm; "Lactose Intolerance," http://www.mayoclinic.org/diseases-conditions/lactose-intolerance/basics/definition/con-20027906.

59 W. Veith and N. Silverberg, "The Association of Acne Vulgaris with Diet," *Cutis* 88, no. 2 (August 2011): 84–91, https://www.ncbi.nlm.nih.gov/pubmed/21916275.

60 P. Cani et al., "Metabolic Endotoxemia Initiates Obesity and Insulin Resistance," *Diabetes* 56, no. 7 (July 2007): 1761–1772, https://www.ncbi.nlm.nih.gov/pubmed/17456850/.

61 P. Cani et al., "Changes in Gut Microbiota Control Metabolic Endotoxemia-Induced Inflammation in High-Fat Diet-Induced Obesity and Diabetes in Mice," *Diabetes* 57, no. 6 (June 2008): 1470–1481, doi: 10.2337/db07-1403, https://www.ncbi.nlm.nih.gov/pubmed/18305141/.

62 "Magnesium," https://ods.od.nih.gov/factsheets/Magnesium-HealthProfessional/.

63 I. Slutsky et al., "Enhancement of Synaptic Plasticity through Chronically Reduced Ca2+ Flux during Uncorrelated Activity," *Neuron* 44, no. 5 (December 2004): 835–849, https://www.ncbi.nlm.nih.gov/pubmed/15572114.

64 A. Mauskop et al., "Intravenous Magnesium Sulfate Relieves Cluster Headaches in Patients with Low Serum Ionized Magnesium Levels," *Headache* 35, no. 10 (November–December 1995): 597–600, https://www.ncbi.nlm.nih.gov/pubmed/8550360.

65 F. Jacka et al., "Association between Magnesium Intake and Depression and Anxiety in Community-Dwelling Adults: The Hordaland Health Study," *Australian and New Zealand Journal of Psychiatry* 43, no. 1 (2009): 45–52, http://www.tandfonline.com/doi/abs/10.1080/00048670802534408.

66 R. Moncayo and H Moncayo, "The WOMED Model of Benign Thyroid Disease: Acquired Magnesium Deficiency Due to Physical and Psychological Stressors Relates to Dysfunction of Oxidative Phosphorylation," *BBA Clinical* 3 (November 12, 2014): 44–64, doi: 10.1016/j.bbacli.2014.11.002, https://www.ncbi.nlm.nih.gov/pubmed/26675817.

67 P. Jakszyn and C. Gonzalez, "Nitrosamine and Related Food Intake and Gastric and Oesophageal Cancer Risk: A Systematic Review of the Epidemiological Evidence," *World Journal of Gastroenterology* 12, no. 27 (July 21, 2006): 4296–4303, https://www.ncbi.nlm.nih.gov/pubmed/16865769; S. Bingham et al., "Does Increased Endogenous Formation of N-Nitroso Compounds in the Human Colon Explain the Association between Red Meat and Colon Cancer?," *Carcinogenesis* 17, no. 3 (March 1996): 515–523, https://www.ncbi.nlm.nih.gov/pubmed/8631138; K. Honikel, "The Use and Control of Nitrate and Nitrite for the Processing of Meat Product," *Meat Science* 78, no. 1–2 (January 2008): 68–76, doi: 10.1016/j.meatsci.2007.05.030, https://www.ncbi.nlm.nih.gov/pubmed/22062097.

Chapter 2: Plant-Based Diets (for Better and Worse)

1 H. Springmann et al., "Analysis and Valuation of the Health and Climate Change Cobenefits of Dietary Change," *Proceedings of the National Academy of Sciences* 113, no. 15 (2016): 4146–4151.

2 J. Powell et al., "Evidence for the Role of Environmental Agents in the Initiation or Progression of Autoimmune Conditions," *Environmental Health Perspectives* 107, suppl. 5 (October 1999): 667–672, https://www.ncbi.nlm.nih.gov/pmc/articles/PMC1566242/.

3 M. Gago-Dominguez et al., "Use of Permanent Hair Dyes and Bladder-Cancer Risk," *International Journal of Cancer* 91, no. 4 (February 2001): 575–579, https://www.ncbi.nlm.nih.gov/pubmed/11251984.

4 C. Cobbett and P. Goldsbrough, "Phytochelatins and Metallothioneins: Roles in Heavy Metal Detoxification and Homeostasis," *Annual Review of Plant Biology* 53 (2002): 159–182, https://www.ncbi.nlm.nih.gov/pubmed/12221971.

5 J. Lamb et al., "A Program Consisting of a Phytonutrient-Rich Medical Food and an Elimination Diet Ameliorated Fibromyalgia Symptoms and Promoted Toxic-Element Detoxification in a Pilot Trial," *Alternative Therapies in Health and Medicine* 17, no. 2 (March–April 2011): 36–44, https://www.ncbi.nlm.nih.gov/pubmed/21717823.

6 P. Tak and G. Firestein, "NF-kB: A Key Role in Inflammatory Diseases," *Journal of Clinical Investigation* 107, no. 1 (January 1, 2001): 7–11, https://www.ncbi.nlm.nih.gov/pmc/articles/PMC198552/.

7 I. Rahman et al., "Regulation of Inflammation and Redox Signaling by Dietary Polyphenols," *Biochemical Pharmacology* 72, no. 11 (November 2006): 1439–1452, https://www.ncbi.nlm.nih.gov/pubmed/16920072.

8 G. Owens and R. Bunge, "Schwann Cells Depleted of Galactocerebroside Express Myelin-Associated Glycoprotein and Initiate but Do Not Continue the Process of Myelination," *Glia* 3, no. 2 (1990): 118–124, https://www.ncbi.nlm.nih.gov/pubmed/1692007.

9 C. Hallert et al., "Increasing Fecal Butyrate in Ulcerative Colitis Patients by Diet: Controlled Pilot Study," *Inflammatory Bowel Diseases* 9, no. 2 (March 2003): 116–121, https://www.ncbi.nlm.nih.gov/pubmed/12769445; A. Di Sabatino et al., "Oral Butyrate for Mildly to Moderately Active Crohn's Disease," *Alimentary Pharmacology and Therapeutics* 22, no. 9 (November 2005): 789–794. https://www.ncbi.nlm.nih.gov/pubmed/16225487.

10 "Diet Rich in Processed Meat 'May Worsen Asthma Symptoms,'" http://www.nhs.uk/news/2016/12December/Pages/Diet-rich-in-processed-meat-may-worsen-asthma-symptoms.aspx.

11 P. Tuso, "Nutritional Update for Physicians: Plant-Based Diets," *Permanente Journal* 17, no. 2 (Spring 2013): 61–66, https://www.ncbi.nlm.nih.gov/pmc/articles/PMC3662288/.

12 H. Vertanen et al., "Intake of Different Dietary Proteins and Risk of Type 2 Diabetes in Men: The Kuopio Ischaemic Heart Disease Risk Factor Study," *British Journal of Nutrition* 117, no. 6 (March 2017): 882–893, doi: 10.1017/S0007114517000745, https://www.ncbi.nlm.nih.gov/pubmed/28397639.

13 A. Vieira et al., "Foods and Beverages and Colorectal Cancer Risk: A Systematic Review and Meta-Analysis of Cohort Studies, an Update of the Evidence of the WCRF-AICR Continuous Update Project," *Annals of Oncology* 28, no. 8 (August 1, 2017): 1788–1802, doi: 10.1093/annonc/mdx171, https://www.ncbi.nlm.nih.gov/pubmed/28407090.

14 A. Perloy et al., "Intake of Meat and Fish and Risk of Head-Neck Cancer Subtypes in the Netherlands

Cohort Study," *Cancer Causes and Control* 28, no. 6 (June 2017): 647–656, doi: 10.1007/s10552-017-0892-0, https://www.ncbi.nlm.nih.gov/pubmed/28382514

15 J. Ranganathan and R. Waite, "Sustainable Diets: What You Need to Know in 12 Charts," World Resources Institute, April 20, 2016. http://www.wri.org/blog/2016/04/sustainable-diets-what-you-need-know-12-charts.

16 Food and Agriculture Organization, *Tackling Climate Change through Livestock: A Global Assessment of Emissions and Mitigation Opportunities* (Rome: FAO, 2013); R. Goodland and J. Anhang, "Livestock and Climate Change. What If the Key Actors in Climate Change Were Pigs, Chickens and Cows?," *World Watch*, November/December 2009; Springmann et al., "Analysis and Valuation of the Health and Climate Change Cobenefits of Dietary Change."

17 "Drawdown: Solutions," http://www.drawdown.org/solutions.

18 http://www.hpj.com/bickel/despite-naysayers-some-follow-savory-path-to-holistic-farming/article_62c97d26-0cf3-11e8-adef-ef0dd43e4388.html.

19 L. Cordain et al., "Origins and Evolution of the Western Diet: Health Implications for the 21st Century," *American Journal of Clinical Nutrition* 81, no. 2 (February 2005): 341–354, http://ajcn.nutrition.org/content/81/2/341.full.

20 A. Di Sabatino et al., "Small Amounts of Gluten in Subjects with Suspected Nonceliac Gluten Sensitivity: A Randomized, Double-Blind, Placebo-Controlled, Cross-Over Trial," *Clinical Gastroenterology and Hepatology* 13, no. 9 (September 2015): 1604-1612.e3, doi: 10.1016/j.cgh.2015.01.029, https://www.ncbi.nlm.nih.gov/pubmed/25701700.

21 E. Luca et al., "Evidence for the Presence of Non-Celiac Gluten Sensitivity in Patients with Functional Gastrointestinal Symptoms: Results from a Multicenter Randomized Double-Blind Placebo-Controlled Gluten Challenge," *Nutrients* 8, no. 2 (February 2016): 84, https://www.ncbi.nlm.nih.gov/pmc/articles/PMC4772047/.

22 P. Cuatrecasas and G. Tell, "Insulin-Like Activity of Concanavalin A and Wheat Germ Agglutinin—Direct Interactions with Insulin Receptors," *Proceedings of the National Academy of Sciences of the USA* 70, no. 2 (February 1973): 485–489, https://www.ncbi.nlm.nih.gov/pmc/articles/PMC433288/.

23 T. Jönsson et al., "Agrarian Diet and Diseases of Affluence—Do Evolutionary Novel Dietary Lectins Cause Leptin Resistance?," *BMC Endocrine Disorders* 5, no. 10 (2005), https://bmcendocrdisord.biomedcentral.com/articles/10.1186/1472-6823-5-10.

24 J. Greger, "Nondigestible Carbohydrates and Mineral Bioavailability," *Journal of Nutrition* 129, no. 7 (July 1, 1999): 1434S–1435S, http://jn.nutrition.org/content/129/7/1434S.full.

25 I. Johnson et al., "Influence of Saponins on Gut Permeability and Active Nutrient Transport In Vitro," *Journal of Nutrition* 116, no. 11 (November 1, 1986): 2270–2277, http://europepmc.org/abstract/MED/3794833/reload=0;jsessionid=lNql0XVFddJUexYpGqH9.2.

26 J. Barrett, "The Science of Soy: What Do We Really Know?," *Environmental Health Perspectives* 114, no. 6 (June 2006): A352–A358, https://www.ncbi.nlm.nih.gov/pmc/articles/PMC1480510/.

27 "Recent Trends in GE Adoption," https://www.ers.usda.gov/data-products/adoption-of-genetically-engineered-crops-in-the-us/recent-trends-in-ge-adoption.aspx.

28 L. Dolan et al., "Naturally Occurring Food Toxins," *Toxins (Basel)* 2, no. 9 (September 2010): 2289–2332, https://www.ncbi.nlm.nih.gov/pmc/articles/PMC3153292/#B73-toxins-02-02289.

29 R. Gupta et al., "Reduction of Phytic Acid and Enhancement of Bioavailable Micronutrients in Food Grains," *Journal of Food Science and Technology* 52, no. 2 (February 2015): 676–684, https://www.ncbi.nlm.nih.gov/pmc/articles/PMC4325021/.

30 L. Pizzorno, "Highlights from the Institute for Functional Medicine's 2014 Annual Conference: Functional Perspectives on Food and Nutrition: The Ultimate Upstream Medicine," *Integrative Medicine (Encinitas)* 13, no. 5 (October 2014): 38–50, https://www.ncbi.nlm.nih.gov/pmc/articles/PMC4684110/.

31 "Fish Oil," https://www.mayoclinic.org/drugs-supplements-fish-oil/art-20364810.

32 B. Davis and P. Kris-Etherton, "Achieving Optimal Essential Fatty Acid Status in Vegetarians: Current Knowledge and Practical Implications," *American Journal of Clinical Nutrition* 78, 3 suppl. (September 2003): 640S–646S, https://www.ncbi.nlm.nih.gov/pubmed/12936959.

33 J. Tur et al., "Dietary Sources of Omega 3 Fatty Acids: Public Health Risks and Benefits," *British Journal of Nutrition* 107 (2012): S23–S52, https://www.cambridge.org/core/services/aop-cambridge-core/content/view/0C287B125293EF075DFF6169154201A6/S0007114512001456a.pdf/dietary_sources_of_omega_3_fatty_acids_public_health_risks_and_benefits.pdf.

34 S. Rosell et al., "Long-Chain n–3 Polyunsaturated

Fatty Acids in Plasma in British Meat-Eating, Vegetarian, and Vegan Men," *American Journal of Clinical Nutrition* 82, no. 2 (August 2005): 327–334, http://ajcn.nutrition.org/content/82/2/327.abstract.

35   W. Craig, "Nutrition Concerns and Health Effects of Vegetarian Diets," *Nutrition in Clinical Practice* 25, no. 6 (December 2010): 613–620, doi: 10.1177/0884533610385707, https://www.ncbi .nlm.nih.gov/pubmed/21139125.

36   U. Ikeda et al., "1,25-Dihydroxyvitamin D3 and All-Trans Retinoic Acid Synergistically Inhibit the Differentiation and Expansion of Th17 Cells," *Immunology Letters* 134, no. 1 (November 2010): 7–16, doi: 10.1016/j.imlet.2010.07.002, https://www.ncbi .nlm.nih.gov/pubmed/20655952.

37   E. Hedrén et al., "Estimation of Carotenoid Accessibility from Carrots Determined by an In Vitro Digestion Method," *European Journal of Clinical Nutrition* 56, no. 5 (May 2002): 425–430, https:// www.ncbi.nlm.nih.gov/pubmed/12001013.

38   F. Watanabe et al., "Vitamin B12-Containing Plant Food Sources for Vegetarians," *Nutrients* 6, no. 5 (May 2014): 1861–1873, https://www.ncbi.nlm.nih .gov/pmc/articles/PMC4042564/#!po=55.8824.

39   W. Hermann et al., "Vitamin B-12 Status, Particularly Holotranscobalamin II and Methylmalonic Acid Concentrations, and Hyperhomocysteinemia in Vegetarians," *American Journal of Clinical Nutrition* 78, no. 1 (July 2003): 131–136, https:// www.ncbi.nlm.nih.gov/pubmed/12816782.

40   C. Keen and M. Gershwin, "Zinc Deficiency and Immune Function," *Annual Review of Nutrition* 10 (1990): 415–431, https://www.ncbi.nlm.nih.gov /pubmed/2200472.

41   K. Simmer and R. Thompson, "Zinc in the Fetus and Newborn," *Acta Paediatrica Scandinavica Supplement* 319 (1985): 158–163, https://www.ncbi.nlm .nih.gov/pubmed/3868917?dopt=Abstract.

42   J. Hunt, "Bioavailability of Iron, Zinc, and Other Trace Minerals from Vegetarian Diets," *American Journal of Clinical Nutrition* 78, no. 3 (September 2003): 633S–639S, http://ajcn.nutrition.org /content/78/3/633S.long.

Chapter 3: The New Keto: Plant-Based Ketogenic Alchemy

1   M. Moriya et al., "Vitamin K2 Ameliorates Experimental Autoimmune Encephalomyelitis in Lewis Rats," *Journal of Neuroimmunology* 170, no. 1–2 (December 2005): 11–20, https://www.ncbi.nlm.nih .gov/pubmed/16146654.

2   S. Schilling et al., "Plasma Lipids and Cerebral Small Vessel Disease," *Neurology* 83, no. 20 (November 2014): 1844–1852, doi: 10.1212 /WNL.0000000000000980, https://www.ncbi .nlm.nih.gov/pubmed/25320101.

3   I. Schatz et al., "Cholesterol and All-Cause Mortality in Elderly People from the Honolulu Heart Program: A Cohort Study."

Chapter 4: Ketotarian Foods: What to Eat and What to Avoid

1   F. De Vadder et al., "Microbiota-Generated Metabolites Promote Metabolic Benefits via Gut-Brain Neural Circuits," *Cell* 156, no. 1–2 (January 16, 2014): 84–96, http://www.cell.com/cell/fulltext /S0092-8674(13)01550-X.

Chapter 6: First Steps: How to Get Started on Your Ketotarian Journey

1   M. Abou-Donia et al., "Splenda Alters Gut Microflora and Increases Intestinal P-Glyocoprotein and Cytochrome P-450 in Male Rats," *Journal of Toxicology and Environmental Health. Part A* 71, no. 21 (2008): 1415–1429, doi: 10.1080 /15287390802328630 http://www.ncbi.nlm.nih .gov/pubmed/18800291

2   "What Are Proteins and What Do They Do?," https://ghr.nlm.nih.gov/primer/howgeneswork /protein.

3   J. Anderson, "Measuring Breath Acetone for Monitoring Fat Loss: Review," *Obesity (Silver Spring)* 23, no. 12 (December 2015): 2327–2334, https://www.ncbi.nlm.nih.gov/pmc/articles /PMC4737348/.

4   Anderson, "Measuring Breath Acetone for Monitoring Fat Loss: Review."

5   P. Urbain, "Monitoring for Compliance with a Ketogenic Diet: What Is the Best Time of Day to Test for Urinary Ketosis?," *Nutrition and Metabolism (London)* 13 (2016): 77, https://www.ncbi.nlm.nih.gov /pmc/articles/PMC5097355/.

6   K. Borer et al., *Medicine and Science in Sports Exercise* 41, no. 8 (August 2009): 1606–1614, doi: 10.1249/MSS.0b013e31819dfe14, https://www.ncbi .nlm.nih.gov/pubmed/19568199.

7   W. Fernando et al., "The Role of Dietary Coconut for the Prevention and Treatment of Alzheimer's Disease: Potential Mechanisms of Action," *British Journal of Nutrition* 114, no. 1 (July 14, 2015): 1–14, doi: 10.1017/S0007114515001452, https:// www.ncbi.nlm.nih.gov/pubmed/25997382.

8   Y. Liu and H. Wang, "Medium-Chain Triglyceride Ketogenic Diet, an Effective Treatment for Drug-Resistant Epilepsy and a Comparison with Other Ketogenic Diets," *Biomedical Journal* 26, no. 1 (January–February 2013): 9–15, doi: 10.4103/2319-4170.107154, https://www.ncbi.nlm.nih.gov/pubmed/23515148

9   M. McCarty and J. DiNicolantonio, "Lauric Acid–Rich Medium-Chain Triglycerides Can Substitute for Other Oils in Cooking Applications and May Have Limited Pathogenicity," *Open Heart* 3, no. 2 (July 27, 2016): e000467, doi: 10.1136/openhrt-2016-000467, https://www.ncbi.nlm.nih.gov/pubmed/27547436.

Chapter 7: Ketotarian Toolboxes: Intermittent Fasting and Other Tips and Tricks

1   M. Harvie et al., "The Effect of Intermittent Energy and Carbohydrate Restriction v. Daily Energy Restriction on Weight Loss and Metabolic Disease Risk Markers in Overweight Women," *British Journal of Nutrition* 110, no. 8 (October 2013): 1534–1547, doi: 10.1017/S0007114513000792, https://www.ncbi.nlm.nih.gov/pubmed/23591120.

2   S. Aly, "Role of Intermittent Fasting on Improving Health and Reducing Diseases," *International Journal of Health Sciences (Qassim)* 8, no. 3 (July 2014): V-VI, https://www.ncbi.nlm.nih.gov/pmc/articles/PMC4257368/.

3   M. Bronwen et al., "Caloric Restriction and Intermittent Fasting: Two Potential Diets for Successful Brain Aging," *Ageing Research Reviews* 5, no. 3 (August 2006): 332–353, doi: 10.1016/; arr. 2006.04.002, https://www.ncbi.nlm.nih.gov/pmc/articles/PMC2622429/.

4   S. Kumar and G. Kaur, "Intermittent Fasting Dietary Restriction Regimen Negatively Influences Reproduction in Young Rats: A Study of Hypothalamo-Hypophysial-Gonadal Axis," *PLoS ONE* 8, no. 1 (2013): e52416, https://doi.org/10.1371/journal.pone.0052416, http://journals.plos.org/plosone/article?id=10.1371/journal.pone.0052416.

5   M. Wei et al., "Fasting-Mimicking Diet and Markers/Risk Factors for Aging, Diabetes, Cancer, and Cardiovascular Disease," *Science Translational Medicine* 9, no. 377 (February 15, 2017): eaai8700, doi: 10.1126/scitranslmed.aai8700.

6   J. Goh et al., "Workplace Stressors & Health Outcomes: Health Policy for the Workplace," https://behavioralpolicy.org/articles/workplace-stressors-health-outcomes-health-policy-for-the-workplace/.

index

blackstrap molasses, 91

blood meter, 121–22

blood sugar. *See also* glucose
grains and, 52–53
lab tests for, 25
plant-based diets and, 49, 81
symptoms of problems with, 25

blueberries, 48, 80, 136, 187

blue-green algae, 99

bok choy, 78, 157, 205

bone broth, 79, 138

BPA (plastic), 46

BrAce. *See* breath acetone

brain
cholesterol and, 34
fats and, 26, 34
inflammation, 129
problems, 14, 34, 66

brain-adrenal axis, 133

brain-derived-neurotrophic
factor (BDNF), 37

brain fog, 36, 65–66, 105

brain-ovary axis, 132

brain-thyroid axis, 134

branched chain amino acid
supplements (BCAAs), 133

brazil nuts, 73

breast milk, 26, 31

breath acetone (BrAce), 22, 122

breath meter, 122

British Medical Journal, 28

broccoli, 47–48, 76–78, 212, 216,
226

broccoli rabe, 243

brown rice syrup, 90

Brussels sprouts, 47, 76–78
recipes, 149, 168, 220, 224

butter, grass-fed, 41, 87

butyrate, 49

c

cabbage, 47, 77–78, 165, 200

cacao nibs, 241

calcium, 40, 42, 61

cancer, 39, 49–50, 130

caraway, 78

carbatarians, 13, 51–53

carbohydrates
adjustments to intake of, 124
cycling, 136–37
finding best level of, 135–37
moderating, 136
net or total, 81
personal needs for, 118–19

carbonated water, 79

Carb Sweet Spot tool, 135–37

cardamom, 78

carrots, 59, 64, 78, 136, 274

casein, 40–41

cashews, 73, 148, 181

catfish, 84, 250

cattle, 50–51

cauliflower, 47, 77–78
recipes, 156, 159–60, 170, 177,
179–81, 184, 199, 221

CDC. *See* Centers for Disease
Control

celery, 78

celiac disease, 32, 53–54

Centers for Disease Control
(CDC), 14

chard, 47, 77–78, 201

chia seeds, 74, 189

Chinese medicine, 93

chives, 78

chlorella (sea vegetable), 47

cholesterol, 27–28, 39, 66, 130

choline, 64, 75

chronic systemic inflammation,
32–34

cilantro, 47, 77, 79

cinnamon, 78

circadian rhythm dysfunction,
133–34

*Clinical Gastroenterology and
Hepatology*, 53

clove, 78

cobamides, 59

cocoa, 235

coconut milk, 79, 181–82, 187,
189, 229, 275

coconut oil, 72, 125

coconut sugar and nectar, 91

cod, 84

coffee, 79

collagen, 64, 114–15

collards, 47, 77–78, 231, 253

conscious breathing, 140

coriander, 78

cortisol (hormone), 133–34

COX-1 (enzyme), 34

COX-2 (enzyme), 34

C-peptide (test), 25, 38

cravings, 17–19, 69, 81, 130

C-reactive protein (CRP), 28, 35

crescendo fasting, 133

Crohn's disease, 49

cross-reactivity labs (tests), 35

CRP (test), 35. *See also*
C-reactive protein

cucumber, 78, 165, 195, 214,
217

cumin, 78

curcumin, 48, 109–10

curry paste, 148

cyclic ketogenic diet (CKD), 30

cytokine IL-10, 33

cytokine model of cognitive
function, 36

d

dairy, 40–41, 87

dark leafy greens, 47, 77

dates, 91

dendritic cells, 65

depression, 14, 36, 66, 83, 102

detoxification
keto flu and, 126–27
pathways, 18, 33
plant-based diet as, 45–48
from technology, 139

DHA. *See* docosahexaenoic acid

diabetes
Alzheimer's as type 3, 38
type 1, 65
type 2, 23–24, 37–38

diets, individual needs in, 63

digestive enzymes, 56, 84

disease. *See* specific diseases
predictors of, 28

docosahexaenoic acid (DHA),
57–58, 66, 83

heart inflammation, 130
heavy metals, 46, 77, 126
heme iron, 60–61
hemp (protein powder), 113, 230
hemp seeds, 74
herbs, 79
herring, 84, 253
Hgb A1C (test), 25, 38
high-fiber diets, 41
high-fructose corn syrup, 89
high-fructose fruit, 87
high-protein ketogenic diet, 30
hippocampus, 38
holy basil (adaptogen), 105
homocysteine, 28, 35
honey, 91
hormones. *See also* individual
    hormones
  healthy fats balancing, 26
  soy and, 55–56
hormone-signaling inflammation,
    130
ho shou wu (adaptogen), 105
hummus, 184
hydration, 124
hydroxyproline (amino acid),
    114
hypochlorhydria (low stomach
    acid), 64
hypothalamic cells, 36
hypothalamic-pituitary-adrenal
    (HPA) axis, 133
hypothalamic-pituitary-gonadal
    (HPG) axis, 132
hypothalamic-pituitary-thyroid
    (HPT) axis, 134

i

IBS. *See* irritable bowel
    syndrome
industrial farming, 52
industrial seed oils, 86
inflammatarians, 51–53
inflammation
  autoimmune diseases and,
    13–15, 32–34, 82
  plant foods and, 47–48

tests for, 35
  types of, 129–30
iNOS pathway, 65, 112
insoluble fiber, 81
Instant Pot, 268–75
insulin, 24, 89
insulin resistance, 24, 53, 90,
    124, 130, 132
interleuken-17, 65
intermittent fasting (IF)
  hormone health and, 132–34
  as Ketotarian tool, 30, 125,
    129–30
  methods of, 131
*International Journal of
    Adolescent Medicine and
    Health*, 16
intestinal gluconeogenesis, 81
intestinal permeability lab
    (test), 35
inulin, 80
iron, 60–61
irritable bowel syndrome (IBS),
    49, 53
isoflavones, 55–56

j

jicama, 78
Journal of Neuroimmunology, 65
*Journal of the American Medical
    Association (JAMA)*, 14, 15

k

kale, 47, 77–78
  recipes, 154–55, 205, 223, 239
kefir, 108
kelp, 78
keto flu, 126–27
ketogenesis, 22
ketogenic diet
  five types of, 29–30
  health benefits of, 31–39
  issues with, 12, 40–43
ketones
  brain and, 36
  as fuel source, 22, 36, 120

increasing, 125
  testing for, 121–23
  types of, 120
ketosis
  adapting metabolism for,
    120–25
  chemistry of, 21–22
  health benefits of, 22–23
  measurement of, 121–23
  seasonal, 137
ketotarian
  definition, 11
Ketotarian diet
  8-week commitment to, 127
  author's experience with,
    66–68
  basic rules of, 85
  beginning, 116–27
  characteristics of, 19
  eating out and, 95–96
  food pyramid of, 85
  food swaps in, 97–98
  meal plans, 278–85
  recipes for, 146–275
  snacks and, 97
  superfoods in, 98–106
  supplements and, 106–12
  toolbox for, 128–43
  variations of, 67–68
  what not to eat in, 86–88
  what to eat in, 71–85
kimchi, 108
kisspeptin (protein), 132
kohlrabi, 78, 250–51
kombu, 78
kombucha, 79, 88, 108
krill oil, 101–2

l

lactose intolerance, 40
lauric acid, 125
LDL cholesterol, 27–28
leaky gut syndrome, 34, 41,
    64, 75
lean body mass (LBM), 76, 119
lectins, 54–55, 74, 88
leeks, 78

about the author

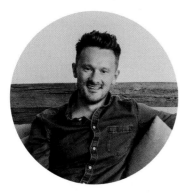

Dr. Will Cole, D.C., IFMCP leading functional-medicine expert, graduated from Southern California University of Health Sciences. His extensive postdoctorate education and training is in functional medicine and clinical nutrition. Dr. Cole consults with people around the world via webcam at drwillcole.com and locally in Pittsburgh, Pennsylvania. He specializes in clinically investigating underlying factors of chronic disease and customizing health programs for thyroid issues, autoimmune conditions, hormonal dysfunctions, digestive disorders, and brain problems.

Dr. Cole was named one of the top fifty functional-medicine and integrative doctors in the nation. A charismatic and popular TV guest frequently called upon to offer advice on health issues, he is a national speaker on functional-medicine topics, and is a health expert and course instructor for mindbodygreen, one of the largest wellness websites in the world, for which he has written hundreds of articles and has a popular video class. Dr. Cole has also written popular articles for goop, Bustle, and *Reader's Digest*.

Dr. Cole has received extensive training in the biological sciences: anatomy, physiology, pathophysiology, epidemiology, histology, blood chemistry, neurology, and pharmacology, as well as conventional medical diagnosis, clinical nutrition, botanical medicine, and lifestyle counseling. He is committed to finding root causes rather than treating symptoms with drugs. His focus is to promote health and optimal function through natural, noninvasive methods such as nutritional therapy, herbs, supplements, stress management techniques, and lifestyle changes.

---

drwillcole.com · **f** **doctorwillcole** · **𝕐** **drwillcole** · **◉** **drwillcole**

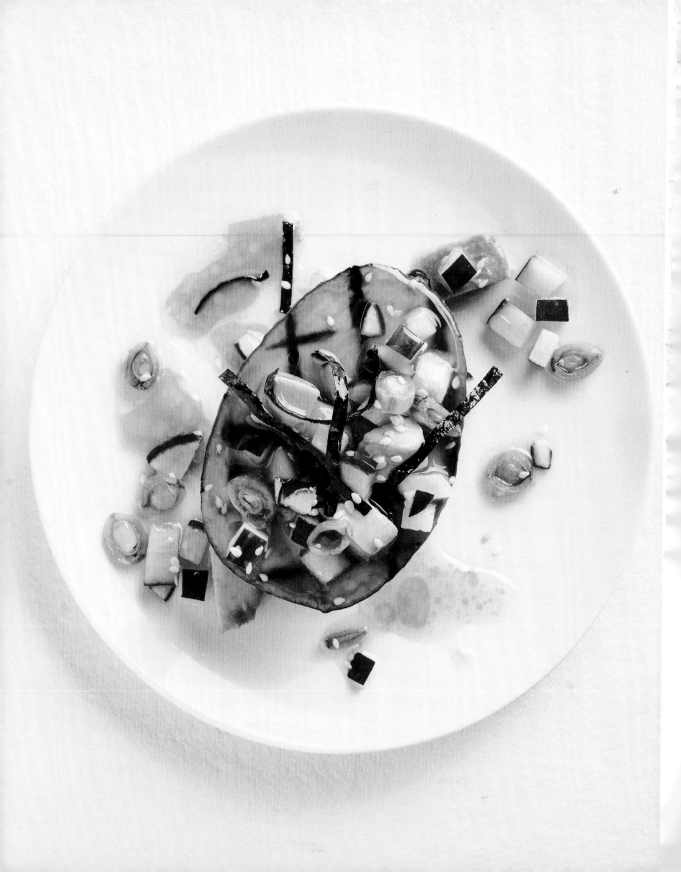